The Biology of Cancer

D0744820

The Biology of Cancer

Second Edition

Edited by
JANICE GABRIEL
MPhil, PgD, BSc(Hons), RN, FETC, ONC, CertMHS
Nurse Director
Central South Coast Cancer Network

John Wiley & Sons, Ltd

Copyright © 2007   John Wiley & Sons Ltd, The Atrium Southern Gate, Chichester,
West Sussex PO19 8SQ, England

Telephone   (+44) 1243 779777

Email (for orders and customer service enquiries): cs-books@wiley.co.uk
Visit our Home Page on www.wiley.com

All Rights Reserved. No part of this publication may be reproduced, stored in a retrieval system or transmitted in any form or by any means, electronic, mechanical, photocopying, recording, scanning or otherwise, except under the terms of the Copyright, Designs and Patents Act 1988 or under the terms of a licence issued by the Copyright Licensing Agency Ltd, 90 Tottenham Court Road, London W1T 4LP, UK, without the permission in writing of the Publisher. Requests to the Publisher should be addressed to the Permissions Department, John Wiley & Sons Ltd, The Atrium, Southern Gate, Chichester, West Sussex PO19 8SQ, England, or emailed to permreq@wiley.co.uk, or faxed to (+44) 1243 770620.

Designations used by companies to distinguish their products are often claimed as trademarks. All brand names and product names used in this book are trade names, service marks, trademarks or registered trademarks of their respective owners. The Publisher is not associated with any product or vendor mentioned in this book.

This publication is designed to provide accurate and authoritative information in regard to the subject matter covered. It is sold on the understanding that the Publisher is not engaged in rendering professional services. If professional advice or other expert assistance is required, the services of a competent professional should be sought.

Other Wiley Editorial Offices

John Wiley & Sons Inc., 111 River Street, Hoboken, NJ 07030, USA

Jossey-Bass, 989 Market Street, San Francisco, CA 94103-1741, USA

Wiley-VCH Verlag GmbH, Boschstr. 12, D-69469 Weinheim, Germany

John Wiley & Sons Australia Ltd, 42 McDougall Street, Milton, Queensland 4064, Australia

John Wiley & Sons (Asia) Pte Ltd, 2 Clementi Loop #02-01, Jin Xing Distripark, Singapore 129809

John Wiley & Sons Canada Ltd, 6045 Freemont Blvd, Mississauga, ONT, L5R 4J3

Wiley also publishes its books in a variety of electronic formats. Some content that appears in print may not be available in electronic books.

Anniversary Logo Design: Richard J. Pacifico

Library of Congress Cataloging in Publication Data

The biology of cancer / edited by Janice Gabriel. — 2nd ed.
   p. ; cm.
  Includes bibliographical references and index.
  ISBN 978-0-470-05759-9 (pbk. : alk. paper)
  1. Cancer. I. Gabriel, Janice.
  [DNLM: 1. Neoplasms—Nurses' Instruction. QZ 200 B6153 2007]
  RC262.B47 2007
  616.99′4—dc22

                            2007012096

British Library Cataloguing in Publication Data

A catalogue record for this book is available from the British Library

ISBN-13: 978-0-470-05759-9

Typeset in 10/12pt Times by Integra Software Services Pvt. Ltd, Pondicherry, India
Printed and bound in Great Britain by TJ International Ltd, Padstow, Cornwall
This book is printed on acid-free paper responsibly manufactured from sustainable forestry in which at least two trees are planted for each one used for paper production.

Contents

CONCORDIA UNIVERSITY LIBRARY
PORTLAND, OR 97211

List of Contributors

David Carpenter
Principal Lecturer, University of Portsmouth

Ailsa Clarke
Lecturer in Biosciences, European Institute of Health and Medical Sciences, University of Surrey

Scott C. Edmunds
Assistant Editor, BioMed Central, London

Francis G. Gabriel
Research Scientist, Translational Oncology Research Centre, Portsmouth Hospitals NHS Trust

Janice Gabriel
Nurse Director, Central South Coast Cancer Network

Louise Knight
Post Doctoral Research Scientist, Translational Oncology Research Centre, Portsmouth Hospitals NHS Trust

Elaine Lennan
Consultant Nurse, Southampton University Hospitals NHS Trust

Helmout Modjtahedi
Visiting Clinical Lecturer, Postgraduate Medical School, University of Surrey

Carmel Sheppard
Consultant Breast Care Nurse, Portsmouth Hospitals NHS Trust/University of Southampton

Debbie Wright
Pharmacist, Central South Coast Cancer Network/Directorate Pharmacist, Southampton University Hospitals NHS Trust Oncology

Preface

Every day we, as cancer nurses, care for patients with life-threatening conditions, and every day we are responsible for the delivery of complex treatments to our patients. We witness at first hand the impact a diagnosis of cancer has for an individual and those around them. We also see how determined our patients are to overcome their diseases. The delivery of treatments to patients in our care necessitates us to have an understanding not only of what they entail, but also of how they work.

The application of biology is playing an ever increasing role in cancer care. There are a number of texts and specialist papers available about the biology of cancer, but they are not, in the main, aimed at cancer nurses, that is the health professionals who actually deliver the majority of treatments. The aim of this book is to be an informative text for students, newly qualified nurses and practising oncology/palliative care nurses. It will also be a useful text for other health care professionals working in the field of cancer, for example radiographers, physiotherapists, dieticians and so on, so that some of the questions asked by patients and their carers can be answered with a clear understanding of what the latest advancements are in the management of an individual's illness.

The aims of this book are:

- To describe what cancer is and its disease process.
- To identify some of the predisposing factors for certain types of cancer.
- To identify the composition of the cell and its functions.
- To discuss the current research and developments relating to biology of cancer.
- To apply the research to the management of an individual patient.
- To summarize current Department of Health guidance to improve access to and quality of cancer care.

Janice Gabriel
March 2007

Acknowledgements

I would like to thank all the contributors to this text, many of whom contributed to the first edition in 2004. I would also like to congratulate those who have recently completed their PhDs, or are about to complete them, and still found time to meet the deadlines for this edition. Without their support and enthusiasm this book would not have been possible.

I would like to dedicate this edition to Imogen and Bethany — the more you learn, the more you grow — and to my colleagues and patients in the Central South Coast Cancer Network.

Janice Gabriel

Acknowledgements

Introduction

Every member of the cancer multidisciplinary team plays a crucial role in the management of their patient. Therefore, each of us has a responsibility to our patients to ensure we have a sound knowledge base, reflecting the latest research and the application of this research to patient care.

This book is written by experienced, practising health care professionals to provide a 'readable' and meaningful text that can easily be applied to patient care. The book is designed not to overwhelm the reader with excessive information on the disease process, but to illustrate how the developments relating to the understanding and application of the biology of cancer can be applied to the management of an individual's care.

The book is divided into three parts, all of which are evidence based and fully referenced. The first part looks at cancer generally and discusses the disease processes, that is the development of a cancer and metastatic spread. It also seeks to identify and explain why there are predisposing factors linked to the development of some cancers, and concludes with a summary of how Department of Health guidance has improved access to cancer services in England.

The second part looks in detail at the cell, its composition, functions and response to cytotoxic agents. It also examines the roles of the immune system and genetics in the development of cancer. This section of the book will also discuss the increasing importance of 'tumour markers' in managing a patient's disease, including their response to treatment.

The final section of the book will tackle the area of research. It takes into account the latest research guidelines, including storage of pathology material, and applies these to patient care so that health care professionals can have a greater understanding of the potential implications for those patients who are considering participating in research studies.

Janice Gabriel

Part I Understanding Cancer

1 What is Cancer?

JANICE GABRIEL

INTRODUCTION

Cancer is not just one disease, but a generic term used to encompass a group of more than two hundred diseases sharing common characteristics. Cancers (carcinomas) are characterized by their unregulated growth and spread of cells to other parts of the body (Corner, 2001; Yarbro, Frogge and Goodman, 2005). Treatment of an individual diagnosed with cancer is not only dependent upon which type of malignancy (cancer) they have, but also on the extent of its spread, together with its sensitivity to treatment (Gabriel, 2001). The total care of the patient will involve assessment of their physical, psychological and social needs, so that a complete care package can be developed to support them and their carer(s) throughout the whole of their patient journey (National Institute for Clinical Excellence (NICE), 2003). (This aspect of care will be further discussed in Chapter 3.)

It is estimated that one in three people in the United Kingdom will develop a malignancy by the time they reach the age of 70, with the incidence increasing with age. This means that approximately 270 000 individuals receive a cancer diagnosis each year in the United Kingdom, with more than 7.5 million affected worldwide (Cornwell, 1997; Department of Health (DoH), 2000a; Corner, 2001). Sadly, as was predicted by Cornwell back in 1997, the UK incidence of cancer is increasing (DoH, 2001a).

This chapter will attempt to provide a clearer understanding of what cancers are and how they spread (metastasize) throughout the body. It will also look at the importance of staging an individual's disease prior to determining the most appropriate management (DoH, 2000a, 2000b).

THE DEFINITION OF CANCER

As humans we are comprised of many millions of cells. Some cells are specific to certain tissues, for example epithelial cells are found throughout the gastrointestinal tract, bladder, lungs, vagina, breast and skin. This group of cells accounts for approximately 70% of cancers (Venitt, 1978; Corner, 2001).

The Biology of Cancer, Second Edition. Edited by J. Gabriel
© 2007 John Wiley & Sons, Ltd.

However, any cell has the potential to undergo malignant changes and lead to the development of a carcinoma. Cancerous cells are not confined to localized 'overgrowth' and infiltration of surrounding tissue, but can spread to other parts of the body via the lymphatic system and bloodstream, creating secondary deposits known as 'metastases' (British Medical Association (BMA), 1997; Walter, 1977; Wells, 2001). This can occur when 'normal' cell control mechanisms become disrupted or indeed fail (Corner, 2001). Surgical removal of the original tumour is not always a successful treatment in malignant disease, due to microscopic spread. Malignant tumours are often irregular in shape, with ill-defined margins (Wolfe, 1986; Walter, 1977). The potential for microscopic spread occurs when the tissue surrounding the visible tumour appears to the eye (macroscopic examination) to be unaffected by cancer. Microscopic examination of the surgical resection margins can reveal the presence of malignant cells. If left untreated, these cells will result in localized recurrence of the cancer and eventual spread (metastasis). The spread of the malignant cells extends outward from the original tumour, and has been described as resembling the appearance of a crab. This is the origin of the term 'cancer', which was derived from the Latin meaning 'crab' (Walter, 1977). The earlier a cancer is detected, the less likely it is to metastasize, and so the more favourable the prognosis for the individual (DoH, 2000a).

METASTATIC SPREAD

All cells replicate themselves. This usually happens about 50−60 times before the cell eventually dies (see Chapter 4) (Corner, 2001; Yarbro, Frogge and Goodman, 2005). However, as malignant cells replicate, they grow in an irregular pattern, infiltrating surrounding tissue. This can result in infiltration of the lymphatics and/or blood vessels. By gaining access to these vessels, malignant cells can be carried to other sites within the patient's body, where they will replicate and grow, rather like rodents establishing colonies in various parts of a town by gaining access to sewer systems (Wolfe, 1986; Walter, 1977). In order to ensure that these malignant cells receive the nourishment they need to thrive, angiogenesis occurs. This is the formation of new blood vessels (Yarbro, Frogge and Goodman, 2005).

Lymphatic Spread

Malignant cells gain access to the lymphatic system and travel along the vessels to the 'regional draining' lymph nodes (Walter, 1977). The malignant cells can then establish residency in these regional nodes, where they replicate and eventually replace the lymph node with a malignant tumour − that is, cancer. Malignant cells from this tumour can then travel, via the lymphatic system, to the next group of lymph nodes, thereby spreading the malignancy throughout the patient's body (Walter, 1977). Lymphomas and squamous cell carcinoma of the head and neck are two examples of where cancer commonly spreads via the lymphatic system (Yarbro, Frogge and Goodman, 2005).

Blood Spread

As with lymphatic spread, malignant cells can also infiltrate the vascular system and travel along the vessels until they arrive at an area where they can become lodged, and subsequently replicate to form a secondary (metastatic) deposit. The malignant cells can then migrate via the smaller blood vessels – that is, the capillaries (Walter, 1977). However, there is evidence that only a small percentage of cells entering the vascular system actually survive to give rise to blood-borne metastatic spread (Walter, 1977). Malignancies which are linked to blood-borne spread include melanoma and small cell carcinoma of the lung (Yarbro, Frogge and Goodman, 2005).

Liver. The commonest site for blood-borne metastases is the liver. Malignancies originating from the gastrointestine, including the pancreas, commonly metastasize to the liver. Other malignancies which can result in secondary deposits in this organ include breast, melanoma, lung and urological cancers (Wolfe, 1986; Walter, 1977).

Lung. The lung is the second most common site for metastatic spread. Tumours that are associated with metastasizing here include the breast, teratomas, melanomas and sarcomas (Wolfe, 1986; Walter, 1977).

Bone. Bone metastases are commonly associated with malignancies of the breast, prostate, kidney, lung and thyroid. Patients with bone metastases can often present with pain. Pathological fractures are not uncommon due to the damage caused to the bone by the malignant cells – that is, the cancer cells replacing the healthy cells and thereby weakening the bone, making it more prone to fracture (Wolfe, 1986; Walter, 1977).

Brain. Brain metastases are closely associated with primary malignancies of the lung, but can also arise from other sites, including the breast, teratomas and malignant melanoma (Wolfe, 1986; Walter, 1977).

Adrenal glands. Breast and lung primary malignancies are more frequently associated with secondary deposits in the adrenal glands, compared to cancers arising from other sites within the body (Wolfe, 1986; Walter, 1977).

Transcoelomic spread. Transcoelomic spread is the term used to describe invasion of the serosal lining of an organ by malignant cells. The malignant cells trigger an inflammatory response, which results in a serous exudate. This is commonly seen in the peritoneal cavity, where it is associated with ovarian and colonic malignancies (Wolfe, 1986; Walter, 1977).

STAGING OF MALIGNANT DISEASE

In order to ensure that a patient can be advised as to the most appropriate management of their particular disease, it is vital that the extent of their cancer is known. For example, if a patient presented with a breast lump, which proved to be malignant, it would be inappropriate to offer the patient a mastectomy if the cancer had already spread to the liver. Removal of the breast would not affect the patient's prognosis, because the cancer had already metastasized at the time of diagnosis. This is why it is so important to 'stage' a patient's cancer before detailed discussions can take place regarding the most appropriate treatment option(s).

The majority of adults with solid tumours are 'staged' using the internationally recognized TNM (tumour, node, metastasis) classification system (UICC, 2002). The TNM classification system was introduced into clinical practice in the early 1950s. It aims to ensure each individual patient is offered the most appropriate treatment for their cancer, depending upon the exact extent of the disease. It also provides an indication of the individual's prognosis, by ensuring that health professionals have standardized information when discussing specific patients' cases and their anticipated responses to treatment, for example at the patient's pre-treatment multi-disciplinary team (MDT) meeting (see Chapter 3). This information will provide a benchmark for future researchers into the treatment of cancer when assessing a patient's disease response against potential new treatments (UICC, 2002; Yarbro, Frogge and Goodman, 2005).

The TNM classification works by assessing the extent of the primary tumour, the involvement of the lymph glands and the presence of metastases (see Table 1.1) (UICC, 2002). A patient diagnosed with a small primary tumour, for example TI,

Table 1.1   TNM classification system.[a]

T = Tumour size	
For example	
T0	No evidence of primary tumour
TI, II, III, IV	Number allocated to size of primary tumour, with 'I' representing the smallest size, up to 'IV', the largest
TX	Primary tumour unable to be assessed
N = Regional lymph node involvement	
For example	
N0	No evidence of regional lymph node involvement
NI, II, III, IV	Number allocated to involvement of regional lymph nodes, ranging from 'I', confined to one group, up to 'IV' when several groups are involved
NX	Regional lymph nodes unable to be assessed
M = Distant metastases	
For example	
M0	No evidence of distant metastatic spread
MI	Evidence of distant metastatic spread
MX	Distant metastasis cannot be assessed

[a] Example only. Not all stages applicable to every cancer.
Source: TNM Classification of Malignant Tumours (2002).

will have a more favourable prognosis than a patient with a large primary tumour and widespread metastases.

The staging process should follow on from the initial diagnostic procedure without any undue delay (DoH, 2000b, 2001, 2004). This can be a tremendously anxious time for the patient and their family members and close friends. The patient has been given a diagnosis of cancer, and will inevitably become concerned about the delay in the commencement of treatment while they wait for further investigations to determine the stage of their disease. A patient whose staging investigations confirm a small primary cancer confined to their larynx may well be successfully treated with radiotherapy, without requiring more radical treatment by laryngectomy. Conversely, a patient with advanced disease which has already metastasized will not have their prognosis improved by undergoing a laryngectomy.

The TNM classification system is commonly used throughout the world for solid tumours, but other classification systems do exist. These include the 'Dukes' staging system for colorectal cancer and the 'Clark's' classification for malignant melanoma. For haematological malignancies, the TNM classifications are not appropriate because of the systemic nature of the diseases. Yarbro, Frogge and Goodman (2005) list a number of classification systems for haematological malignancies, including:

- Ann Arbor classification for lymphomas
- French, American, British (FAB) classification for myeloblastic leukaemia
- Rai classification for chronic lymphocytic leukaemia.

DIAGNOSTIC AND STAGING INVESTIGATIONS

Today, a growing number of tests can be performed to identi abnormal cells or an abnormal structure. These tests can simply c a primary cancer (diagnose), or they can help determine the spread of the malignancy (stage). Essentially these investigations fall into three main groups:

1. Radiology
2. Pathology
3. Endoscopy.

RADIOLOGY

Radiology allows for visualization of the internal structures. Images are created, which the radiologist then interrupts. These images can be created in a number of ways:

X-rays. X-rays or gamma rays are passed through a particular part of the body to generate an image, for example a chest X-ray or mammogram (Yarbro, Frogge and

Goodman, 2005). In order to achieve a clearer image, especially in the gastrointestinal tract, lymphatic vessels, urinary tract and so on, a contrast medium can be used. This involves injecting or, in the case of gastrointestinal studies, asking the patient to swallow a contrast medium. These contrast medium enhances the structures, thereby providing clinicians with more detailed information (Yarbro, Frogge and Goodman, 2005).

Computerized axial tomography (CAT or CT scan). This is an X-ray technique which involves taking a series of X-rays in 'slices'. The images are then analysed by a computer to produce a three-dimensional picture.

Magnetic resonance imaging (MRI). Magnetic resonance imaging does not involve the patient or staff being exposed to ionizing radiation. The patient lies on a couch within a powerful magnetic field and the field aligns the patient's hydrogen nuclei in one direction. Pulses of radio waves are used to disturb the magnetized nuclei and change their alignment. This results in images being generated, which are captured and analysed by a computer. This procedure is excellent for generating detailed images, especially of soft tissue structures. The procedure from the patient's perspective is not dissimilar to undergoing a CT scan (Yarbro, Frogge and Goodman, 2005).

Ultrasound. Ultrasound involves the use of high frequency sound waves. The sound waves are directed over a particular area of the patient's body, via a probe rubbed over the skin, and echoes are 'bounced back'. These echoes can be interpreted to provide information relating to the density of the underlying structures. This is particularly useful in distinguishing cysts from more solid structures (Yarbro, Frogge and Goodman, 2005).

Nuclear medicine imaging. Nuclear medicine imaging involves the parenteral or enteral administration of radioactive compounds. The radioactive material concentrates in the organs or tissues under investigation. A special camera (gamma camera) is used to obtain images of the specific organ/tissues, for interpretation by the radiologist.

Positron emission tomography (PET). Biochemical compounds, 'tagged' with radioactive particles, are administered to the patient. Images are obtained based on the biochemical and metabolic activity of the tissue, and are interpreted by the radiologist (Yarbro, Frogge and Goodman, 2005).

PATHOLOGY

Pathology tests can confirm a clinical diagnosis, and have been used recently to monitor a patient's disease and response to treatment (see Chapter 9). The types of pathology tests that can be undertaken include:

Biochemistry. Body fluids such as blood, urine and so on can be used to identify values that fall outside the range expected in a 'healthy' individual. For example, an elevated bilirubin and alkaline phosphatase could be indicative of liver disease. A raised calcium could indicate bone metastases (Yarbro, Frogge and Goodman, 2005).

Monoclonal antibodies. The production of monoclonal antibodies can lead to the detection of specific tumour antigens, such as HER2 in one type of breast cancer (see Chapter 10) (Cook *et al.*, 2001).

Tumour markers. Tumour markers are proteins, antigens, genes or enzymes that can be produced by a tumour. Testing body fluids, including blood, for these markers can be useful in reaching a diagnosis or monitoring an individual's disease (see Chapter 9).

Biopsy. A biopsy provides tissue for histological examination (Yarbro, Frogge and Goodman, 2005).

Cytology. Cytology involves looking at cells which have been obtained from fluid, secretions, washings from irrigation of cavities, or brushing from tissues (Yarbro, Frogge and Goodman, 2005).

ENDOSCOPY

Endoscopy involves the passage of a long flexible bundle of fibreoptic lights. Images are reflected back to the head of the endoscope, providing the operator with a clear picture of the tissues/organs being examined. It is possible for the operator to obtain samples of tissue for histological examination. A pair of special forceps is passed through the endoscope to the area requiring biopsy. The tissue is then retrieved through the endoscope and sent to the laboratory. Cells for cytological examination can also be obtained via this method.

CONCLUSION

Cancer comprises a complex group of diseases, which currently affect one in three people in the United Kingdom. Successful treatment is dependent not only upon advances in medical science, but also on early detection of the disease, careful staging to determine the extent of the cancer at the time of diagnosis, prompt treatment and appropriate support for the patient.

2 Predisposing Factors to Developing Cancer

JANICE GABRIEL

INTRODUCTION

As society becomes more affluent, so the incidence of cancer can be demonstrated to rise. There could be a number of explanations for this, including increased wealth and longevity (Gabriel, 2001; Richards, 2006). People are surviving previously life-threatening incidents, such as infectious diseases, major accidents and so on, only to live longer and potentially go on to develop cancer later in life. We know that more affluent societies consume higher amounts of convenience foods, alcohol and tobacco, and the United Kingdom is certainly no exception to this observation. We in the West are exposed to higher levels of chemicals and pollutants than people living in many less developed parts of the world. These factors can contribute to an individual developing a malignancy (Venitt, 1978; Corner, 2001; Richards, 2006). Other factors include past exposure to ionizing radiation and viruses, and a genetic disposition (Yarbro, Frogge and Goodman, 2005). However, having a genetic disposition does not automatically mean that an individual will go on to develop a particular cancer (see Chapter 7).

This chapter will look at the possible links between specific cancers and the lifestyles people adopt and the environments in which they live. It will also identify the steps which are being taken to minimize the risks and identify cancers at an earlier stage.

HISTORICAL PERSPECTIVE

As long ago as 1775, Percival Pot, a London surgeon, described the link between cancer of the scrotum and employment as a chimney sweep (Walter, 1977). Pot observed that there was a higher incidence of carcinoma of the scrotum in young boys who worked sweeping chimneys than in those employed in other occupations – the earliest described occupationally acquired malignancy. Although not designed as a scientific study to establish the cause of cancer in this group of boys, a causal link was identified.

The Biology of Cancer, Second Edition. Edited by J. Gabriel
© 2007 John Wiley & Sons, Ltd.

In 1896, a German physicist, Roentgen, identified the use of radiation (X-rays) as a diagnostic tool. Further research into the uses of radiation resulted in it being used as an innovative treatment for cancer by the close of the nineteenth century. However, within seven years of Roentgen's discovery, a causal link between exposure to radiation and the development of leukaemia was established (Yarbro, Frogge and Goodman, 2005).

An early laboratory experiment, undertaken in 1915, proved for the first time that it was possible to develop cancer as a direct result of exposure to a chemical. The chemical was coal tar. The experiment involved applying coal tar to the skin of a rabbit, resulting in the rabbit developing skin cancer (Yarbro, Frogge and Goodman, 2005).

Horton-Taylor (2001) wrote about the study undertaken by Doll and Hill in the 1950s, looking at the incidence of lung cancer among British doctors. This study established a link between smoking and the development of small cell (oat cell) carcinoma of the lung. Further work undertaken by Doll and Hill identified that risk of dying from lung cancer is 32 times higher in heavy smokers than in non-smokers (Horton-Taylor, 2001). There is now a proven link between cigarette smoking and the development of lung cancer later in life. The evidence is so overwhelming that the UK government has included smoking cessation as one of its targets, which is supported by strong advertising campaigns and health education programmes (DoHa, 2001; Richards, 2006).

At the beginning of the twenty-first century, we have come a long way since Pot's chance observation of cancer of the scrotum in chimney sweep boys. Studies are now scientifically designed and undertaken specifically to identify causal links between exposure to certain substances and the development of cancer (see Chapters 12 and 13).

DIET

COLORECTAL CANCER

Back in 1978, Gillis and Holes highlighted a link between a low-fibre diet and carcinoma of the large bowel. Today it is well recognized that a diet that is low in fibre and high in animal fats can significantly contribute to the development of colorectal cancer (Cartmel and Reid, 2000; Yarbro, Frogge and Goodman, 2005). The consumption of five portions of fresh fruit and vegetables each day has been demonstrated to decrease the risk of developing this type of cancer in later life (DoH, 2000a). *The NHS Cancer Plan* (DoH, 2000a) advocates increasing the daily consumption of fresh fruit and vegetables to reduce the risk of developing cancer. Indeed, as part of a national health promotion campaign, children attending infant schools in England are now provided with a portion of fresh fruit at their morning break.

It is estimated that a third of all cancers − and possibly as many as 90% of colorectal malignancies − are directly linked to diet (Yarbro, Frogge and

Goodman, 2005). In the United Kingdom, 25 000 individuals are diagnosed with colorectal cancer each year, and the incidence is increasing (Harrocopus and Myers, 1996; Richards, 2006). The majority of those affected by this disease, that is 75%, will be in excess of 65 years, with a median age of 70 (Yarbro, Frogge and Goodman, 2005).

The incidence of colorectal cancer in the United Kingdom is (Whittaker, 2001):

- 4 per 100 000 under 50 years
- 100 per 100 000 in 50−69 year olds
- 300 per 100 000 over 70 years.

If a patient develops a cancer, the prognosis is improved if it can be detected early, and colorectal malignancies are no exception. In the late summer of 2006, the DoH introduced a national bowel screening programme for individuals aged between 60 and 69. This involves people collecting three samples of their stools on specially provided test strips and sending the samples back to a regional testing centre via post. Those individuals who test positively for occult blood in their samples will be contacted and invited to attend for further investigations. By October 2006, the screening programme had already identified a percentage of the screening population with cancer, that is people who had no idea they had bowel cancer (Richards, 2006).

BREAST CANCER

The development of cancer through dietary factors is not confined to colorectal malignancies. In 1975 a study by Armstrong and Doll identified a diet high in fats as a possible contributing cause to the development of breast cancer (Willett, 1989; Sheppard, 2001). However, Yarbro, Frogge and Goodman (2005) suggest that the consumption of fat alone is not a contributing cause, and identify rather the total number of calories consumed, especially those consumed in early life.

In the United Kingdom, the incidence of breast cancer is increasing. In the 1970s it was estimated to affect 1 in 17 of the female population, but by 2006 it had risen to 1 in 11 (Richards, 2006).

STOMACH CANCER

In Japan there is a high incidence of stomach cancer. It is more common than other types of malignancy in that country. Yet, when Japanese people move to the United States, it has been observed that the incidence of stomach cancer reduces, and the incidences of breast and colorectal malignancies increase in line with the indigenous population. This was highlighted by Willett (1989) as being directly attributable to change in diet − that is, the Japanese had abandoned/reduced their former diets, which contained high amounts of salted fish, in favour of a more Western diet that is high in fat and low in fibre.

TOBACCO/SMOKING

There is overwhelming evidence to link tobacco with a variety of cancers. While smoking unquestionably contributes significantly to the development of small cell (oat cell) carcinoma of the lung and bladder cancer, it must not be forgotten that it can be consumed in a variety of different ways (Yarbro, Frogge and Goodman, 2005). These include chewing, sniffing and inhalation from passive smoking. The malignant conditions linked to the use of/exposure to tobacco include (Horton-Taylor, 2001):

* small cell (oat cell) carcinoma of the lung
* oropharnygeal cancer
* bladder cancer
* cervical cancer
* gastric cancer
* lip cancer
* pancreatic cancer.

LUNG CANCER

Lung cancer is now one of the commonest malignancies affecting both men and women in the United Kingdom (Horton-Taylor, 2001). Although its incidence is decreasing in males, it is still rising in the female population (Gillis, 1978; Richards, 2006). This is not a pattern unique to the United Kingdom, as the incidence of smoking related lung cancers is not expected to peak among American women until 2010 (Yarbro, Frogge and Goodman, 2005). Studies in both the United States and the United Kingdom indicate that despite the publicity linking cigarette smoking and cancer, the incidence of lung cancer is continuing to rise, especially in females from lower socioeconomic groups (Gillis, 1978; Yarbro, Frogge and Goodman, 2005). The UK government is well aware of the huge part smoking plays in the development of cancers. *The NHS Cancer Plan* (DoH, 2000a) aims to reduce smoking in adults, from 28% to 24% by 2010, by developing local targeted action. This includes the provision of services to help individuals quit smoking, the availability of nicotine replacement therapy – on prescription since April 2001 – and legislation to create smoke-free public areas, for example bars and restaurants, by the summer of 2007 in England (DoH, 2001a; Richards, 2006).

PASSIVE SMOKING

Passive smoking is linked to the development of cancer among non-smokers. There have been a number of litigation cases in the United States, where compensation has been paid to individuals diagnosed with smoking related malignancies who have involuntarily shared office space with smokers for many years (Fielding and Phenow, 1988).

In the United Kingdom advertising campaigns to raise awareness of the potential dangers of passive smoking have been launched by the government, including a successful television campaign identifying the effects on children. In July 2007, legislation was enforced to ban smoking indoors in all public areas in England (Northern Ireland, Wales and Scotland already have such a ban in place) (Richards, 2006).

ORAL CANCER

In India, cancer of the oral cavity accounts for a high percentage of all malignancies registered annually. This malignancy is linked to the social habit of chewing quids of betel, lime and tobacco. The constant irritation to the tissues of the cheek and gum can lead to an individual developing an oral malignancy over time (Gillis, 1978).

BLADDER CANCER

Smoking was first linked to the development of bladder cancer in the mid-1950s (Lind and Hagan, 2000). Studies have identified that 50% of bladder cancers may be attributable to smoking (Gillis, 1978; Lind and Hagan, 2000).

VIRUSES

Early work looking at the link between viruses and the development of cancers has led to the discovery of human genes associated with cancer (Yarbro, Frogge and Goodman, 2005) (see Chapters 6 and 7). One example of viral exposure linked to a malignancy is hepatitis B in liver cancer (Hausen, 1991; Yarbro, Frogge and Goodman, 2005). However, there are a number of other viruses linked to specific cancers and these include:

- HTLV-1   T-cell lymphoma and T-cell leukaemia
- HTLV-2   Hairy-cell leukaemia
- Epstein-Barr virus   Burkitt's lymphoma
- Hepatitis C virus   Liver cancer
- Human papilloma virus Cervical cancer.

To attempt to reduce the incidence of cervical cancer, research has resulted in the development of vaccines for the human papilloma virus. However, any vaccination would have to take place before a girl became sexually active to maximize its effectiveness (Richards, 2006).

BACTERIA

Helicobacter pylori can live in the lining of the stomach and is linked to the development of gastric and duodenal ulcers. It is now known that there is a link between chronic ulcer disease and the development of malignancy. This bacterium can be eradicated by treatment with antibiotics, reducing the risk of developing gastric cancer in the future (Yarbro, Frogge and Goodman, 2005).

RADIATION

Today it is well recognized that exposure to radiation can have a carcinogenic effect on living cells. Ionizing radiation releases enough energy to damage the DNA within each cell, which can result in malignant changes taking place in later life. Exposure can be in the form of repeated doses or one isolated incident, such as the radiation victims at Chernobyl in 1986 (Walter, 1977; Yarbro, Frogge and Goodman, 2005).

The most common forms of radiation induced cancers are basal cell carcinoma and squamous carcinoma of the skin. These can arise from excessive exposure to ultraviolet radiation (UVR) − that is, the sun (Yarbro, Frogge and Goodman, 2005). The use of radiation in medicine and industry is now closely controlled, with the specified maximum annual doses for each individual closely monitored (Palmer, 2001). Over time, and with increasing knowledge of the potential dangers of ionizing radiation, these annual doses have been reduced (Palmer, 2001). Exposure to ionizing radiation can result in the following malignancies:

- leukaemia
- thyroid cancer
- squamous cell carcinoma of the skin.

ASBESTOS

Exposure to asbestos is now known to be responsible for causing mesothelioma. Up until the 1970s, asbestos was widely used in the UK building industry. The asbestos, in the form of a fine, white powder, was inhaled by staff handling the material. The onset of the resulting malignancy, that is mesothelioma, could run over a period of many years from the initial exposure. The use of asbestos has now been greatly reduced. When it is handled, for example in the demolition of buildings, staff exposure is closely monitored, with strict enforcement in the provision of protective clothing (Yarbro, Frogge and Goodman, 2005).

Table 2.1 Chemicals/agents linked to specific cancers

Chemical/Agent	Cancer
Asbestos	Mesothelioma
Pitch, soot, coal tar, oil	Squamous cell carcinoma of the skin, scrotum
Vinyl chloride	Liver
Arsenic	Sinuses, lung
Benzidine	Bladder
Wool/leather/wood dust	Nasal sinuses
Aniline dyes	Bladder

CHEMICALS

A number of chemicals, if not handled correctly, can be linked to the development of cancer in later life (these are summarized in Table 2.1). Where occupational exposure is unavoidable, legislation exists to ensure that exposure is minimized and the health of individuals is closely monitored (Yarbro, Frogge and Goodman, 2005).

POLLUTION

As our society becomes more affluent, so we consume more and generate increasing waste products, leading to pollution. Our increasing use of chlorofluorocarbons (CFCs) is leading to the destruction of the ozone layer, resulting in more ultraviolet radiation reaching the earth. This is a contributing factor to the increase in the number of skin cancers.

GENETICS

With the development of molecular biology, new techniques are leading to the identification of genes which increase an individual's predisposition to develop cancer (see Chapter 7). Genes already identified include (Yarbro, Frogge and Goodman, 2005):

- RBI   Retinoblastoma
- WT1   Wilm's tumour
- APC   Familial polyposis
- CDKN2   Dysplastic nevus syndrome
- FACC   Fanconi's anaemia
- BLM   Bloom syndrome (associated with leukaemia)
- BRCA1   Breast and ovarian cancer
- BRCA2   Breast cancer.

Back in 1984, Lynch and Alban believed that as many as 15% of all cancers had a genetic link (Yarbro, Frogge and Goodman, 2005). However, with advances in medical science, including the human genome project, this estimate may be revised as new knowledge is acquired (see Chapter 7). We already know that genetic damage by such substances as tobacco, radiation and so on can lead to gene mutation. Damaged (mutated) genes can then lead to an individual developing cancer (see Chapters 4 and 7).

THE NHS CANCER PLAN

In September 2000, *The NHS Cancer Plan* was published by the DoH (2000a). This publication had four main aims:

1. to save more lives;
2. to ensure people with cancer get the right professional support and care as well as the best treatments;
3. to tackle the inequalities in health that mean unskilled workers are twice as likely to die from cancer as professionals; and
4. to build for the future through investment in the cancer workforce, through strong research and through preparation for the genetics revolution, so that the NHS never falls behind in cancer care again.

This document identifies the government's strategy for tackling cancer. Not only has cancer been made one of the main priorities within the NHS; for the first time a cohesive approach to care has been employed throughout the entire patient journey: primary, secondary and tertiary care, working with the voluntary sector and consumers of health care, that is patients and carers, to develop effective programmes for prevention, diagnosis, treatment, supportive care and research (DoH, 2000a). *The NHS Cancer Plan* (DoH, 2000a) set out clear objectives for providers of cancer services to meet, to ensure that all patients have access to speedier diagnostic services and treatments. By 2001, all patients who were suspected of having a possible cancer, when they consulted their general practitioner (GP), were referred to the appropriate hospital specialist and seen within two weeks. Hospitals are now required to monitor such referrals to ensure that if breaches in the waiting times do occur, appropriate actions are taken to rectify the problem. Today, a patient who is referred as having a suspected cancer is actively 'tracked' during their investigative stage to ensure that they wait no longer than 62 days from urgent referral by their general practitioner, to commencing their treatment. For those patients who are not referred urgently, but are subsequently identified as having a malignancy, a national target has been set to ensure their treatment commences within 31 days of their diagnosis. By August 2006, 95 % of patients on both the 31- and 62-day pathways commenced their treatment within the targets (Richards, 2006).

HEALTH PROMOTION

The development of cancers can be a result of lifestyles adopted over many years. Health promotion needs to start at an early age in order to have maximum effect in reducing an individual's risk of developing cancer in later life. It has already been said that as many as a third of all cancers are linked to diet, with a further third linked to smoking (DoH, 2000a; Yarbro, Frogge and Goodman, 2005). By working closely with health promotion departments and primary care, the UK government intends to continue to reduce the incidence of smoking. This is to be achieved by (DoH, 2000a; Richards, 2006):

• banning tobacco advertising;
• developing NHS provided smoking cessation services;
• providing nicotine replacement therapy on prescription;
• enforcing the law to prohibit the sale of cigarettes to children under 16;
• establishing a smoking cessation helpline; and
• introducing legislation to ban smoking in enclosed public areas.

To raise the awareness of the importance of the consumption of fresh fruit and vegetables, the government is committed to working closely with the food industry and the Food Standards Agency (DoH, 2000a). The overall intention is to increase the availability and affordability of fresh fruit and vegetables to all members of society, with a recommendation that at least five pieces/portions should be consumed each day. One initiative includes 'The National School Fruit Scheme'. This scheme aims to ensure that all children aged between four and six receive a free piece of fruit each day at school (DoH, 2000a).

Other health promotion campaigns are aimed at raising awareness of the link between heavy alcohol consumption and the development of cancer, as well as the dangers of inappropriate protection from sunlight, the need to reduce obesity and the importance of regular physical activity (DoH, 2000a).

HEALTH SCREENING

It is important to understand the difference between 'screening' and 'testing'. Screening is intended to look at large numbers of asymptomatic individuals in an attempt to identify a potential underlying problem at an early stage. Testing is a specific intention to find out the cause of an individual's symptoms. Individuals included in screening programmes tend to have generalized characteristics, for example they fall into a specific age band or are of the same sex. Since 2004 all women aged between 50 and 70 have been included in the national breast screening programme in the United Kingdom (DoH, 2000a). Screening investigations should be minimally invasive and not too uncomfortable, in order to ensure maximum take-up by the target population. A diagnostic test is a deliberate attempt to identify the cause of an individual's symptoms. If someone has a positive screening result they will inevitably be advised to undergo further investigations, for example those individuals who screen positive for occult blood in their stool samples as part of the national bowel screening programme. In these cases more invasive, diagnostic tests may well be suggested to determine the cause of the abnormality, for example colonoscopy (Gabriel, 2001; Richards, 2006).

BREAST SCREENING

The breast screening programme was launched in the United Kingdom in 1988. Now, all women aged between 50 and 70 are invited to undergo breast screening mammography every three years (DoH, 2000a). Those who have an abnormality detected by the screening mammography are 'recalled' to the screening centre and undergo further investigations.

CERVICAL SCREENING

In 1988, a national cervical screening programme was established in the United Kingdom for all women aged between 20 and 64. Since its introduction, the death rate from cervical cancer has been reducing year on year (DoH, 2000a). The screening technique originally involved taking a sample of cells from the cervix and applying them to a slide. This is currently being replaced by a technique known as 'liquid-based cytology', which is a more reliable method of obtaining a satisfactory sample for screening (Richards, 2006).

Although vaccines have been developed against the human papilloma virus (the commonest cause of cervical cancer), they are not yet widely available. Even when they do become more widely used, for example as part of a possible vaccination programme, the cervical screening programme will need to continue for many more years to take account of women who have already been exposed to the virus (Richards, 2006).

PROSTATE SCREENING

Some men diagnosed with prostate cancer have elevated levels of prostate-specific antigen (PSA). There is also a significant percentage of men with an elevated PSA who do not have prostate cancer. As yet, not enough is known about the possible links between an elevated PSA and prostate cancer to enable a screening programme to be developed based on the PSA blood test alone. There is currently ongoing research in this area (see Chapter 9).

COLORECTAL SCREENING

There is strong evidence to link the early detection and treatment of colorectal cancer to improved survival rates. In the summer of 2006, the phased roll out of the national bowel screening programme in the United Kingdom commenced to include 60–69 year olds (Richards, 2006).

OVARIAN SCREENING

Currently two possible techniques are being evaluated as potential screening methods for ovarian cancer. These include trans-vaginal ultrasound and a blood test for the antigen CA125 (see Chapter 9) (DoH, 2000a).

EARLY DETECTION

While reducing the risks associated with the development of cancer plays a key role in reducing the overall incidence of the disease, the next biggest challenge is to be able to identify the disease at an earlier stage. The results of research and advances in technology are playing vital roles here. The 31- and 62-day targets are also having a positive impact on the speed of patients' diagnoses and initial treatments, but more still needs to be done. Through the publication of *The NHS Cancer Plan* (DoH, 2000a) and the 2005 DoH guidance on referrals for suspected cancer, health professionals have worked with their Primary Care Trusts (PCTs) to develop guidance for GPs on the referral criteria for patients with clinical features which could be suggestive of an underlying malignancy. Patients referred under this mechanism are now fast tracked to see an appropriate specialist. These patients should wait no longer than fourteen calendar days from the time they consult their GP until their hospital consultation. These patients are also prioritized to undergo diagnostic tests, ensuring a diagnosis is reached without any inappropriate delays. However, only a third of patients who ultimately receive a diagnosis of cancer currently commence their patient journey as an urgent GP referral, that is, are suspected initially of having symptoms which could be cancer (Richards, 2006).

CONCLUSION

The incidence of cancer is increasing for a variety of reasons: lifestyles, increasing age of the population and so on. More streamlined approaches to care, especially in relation to effective screening programmes, prompt referral, investigation, early detection and treatment, should ultimately see a decrease in the overall mortality associated with this group of diseases. The benefits of research will not only be advantageous to those affected by the disease, but to society as a whole. New genetic tests and future research will hopefully be able to influence the development of cancer for future generations. However, this will come with a financial price tag and hard decisions will have to be made.

3 Cancer: What Does a Diagnosis Mean for an Individual and What Are the Implications for Society?

JANICE GABRIEL

INTRODUCTION

Every year in the United Kingdom, 270 000 individuals are diagnosed with cancer, with a further 120 000 dying in England alone as a direct result of this group of diseases (Cornwell, 1997; DoH, 2000a). It is currently estimated that one in three people in the United Kingdom will develop a malignancy by the age of 70, with the incidence rising. This equates to 700 individuals each day, in England, receiving a diagnosis of cancer (DoH, 2000a; Richards, 2006).

This chapter discusses some of the issues that a diagnosis of cancer can raise for an individual, their family and friends. It also outlines the government's efforts to improve the standard of cancer services, and what this means for patients embarking on their 'cancer journey' today.

A DIAGNOSIS OF CANCER

Cancer is a protracted illness, always raising uncertainty in the minds of those affected, and their family and friends, as to whether the disease can be successfully treated. Historically, the management of an individual with cancer has revolved around medically led models of care — that is, investigation, diagnosis, treatment and follow-up/palliative care. However, health professionals and government policy are beginning to 're-think' cancer, and move it into the chronic group of diseases. This is a consequence of more individuals living longer after their initial diagnosis and receiving various forms of treatment to control their cancer and alleviate its symptoms (Richards, 2006).

The treatment of cancer is not just about treating the disease. Behind every cancer diagnosis there is a person. Although some efforts have been made in the past to address the holistic needs of patients and their families, it is only recently that there

The Biology of Cancer, Second Edition. Edited by J. Gabriel
© 2007 John Wiley & Sons, Ltd.

has been national guidance − resulting in national standards, which are contained in the *Manual for Cancer Services* (DoH, 2000a, 2000b; Whittaker and Sheppard, 2001; Young, 2001; DoH, 2004; Richards, 2006).

As discussed earlier in this book, cancer is a group of diseases, with some forms of malignancy, such as basal cell carcinoma of the skin, carrying an excellent prognosis for the patient (NICE, 2005; Yarbro, Frogge and Goodman, 2005; Wheeler, 2006). However, as health professionals we must not be complacent when using the word 'cancer'. It is important that the diagnosis is imparted to the patient, and their families and carers, with tact and adequate explanation of its potential implications, even if theirs is a form of the disease that responds well to treatment (DoH, 2000a; Young, 2001; Wheeler, 2006). Cancer instils fear in most individuals affected. Many patients, together with their family and friends, experience feelings of uncertainty about their future. Young (2001) discusses how patients want honest and positive answers. Is the disease treatable? If so, what will the treatment involve − surgery, radiotherapy, chemotherapy? What is the likelihood of the success of the treatment? Will they be cured? Will the cancer, or indeed the treatment, result in any adverse effects in the future? What is the risk of the cancer returning? Is there any inherited risk with this type of cancer? If the cancer is untreatable, what can be done? What does the future hold? What are the financial implications for the patient and their family? Will the cancer affect the relationship between the patient and his or her partner?

We all find bad news distressing, but how we react depends on our personalities and circumstances. Young (2001) discusses how some individuals experience the 'grief' process at different stages, for example when they embark on the investigation trail for a possible diagnosis of cancer, or when they are given the diagnosis of cancer. It is not only the patient who requires time and support, but also their family and friends for the entire patient journey − a journey that is unique for every individual and carer (DoH, 2000a; Wheeler, 2006).

The NHS Cancer Plan (DoH, 2000a) stresses the importance of good communication between health professionals and patients. But, however good communication is, it alone is insufficient. The individual patient, together with carers and family members, needs the offer of ongoing support from the time of diagnosis and throughout the entire patient journey. If the offer is initially refused, health professionals need to ensure that it is repeated at appropriate times. Support can take the form of active listening, providing written information, or onward referral to other professionals, such as specialist nurses, social workers, palliative care specialists, counselling services, voluntary organizations and so on. Whatever support is offered, it must be appropriate for that individual (Young, 2001).

The NHS Cancer Plan (DoH, 2000a, p. 64) summarizes some surveys of cancer patients, identifying that patients give great importance to:

• Being treated with humanity − with dignity and respect
• Good communication with health professionals
• Being given clear information about their condition

- Receiving the best possible symptom control
- Receiving psychological support when they need it.

Each patient is a unique individual, and as such we as health professionals must respond to their individual requirements, irrespective of their social, cultural or religious background. We should not raise unrealistic expectations, but at the same time we must be honest, yet sensitive to the content of our discussions. For most patients, they are embarking on a long and complex journey − a journey for which no one can guarantee the outcome − a journey that is unique to them.

THE NHS CANCER PLAN

Back in 1995, a document was published by the DoH known as *A Framework for Commissioning Cancer Services,* commonly referred to as the 'Calman−Hine Report' (DoH, 1995). This document recommended the establishment of specialist cancer networks. These networks were to be responsible for coordinating the care provided in primary, secondary and tertiary care, to ensure that all individuals receive equity of access to services and a uniformly high standard of cancer care, delivered by a skilled and knowledgeable cancer workforce. Today there are 33 cancer networks in England (DoH, 1995).

Following on from the publication of the Calman−Hine Report (Richards, 2006), *The NHS Cancer Plan* (DoH, 2000a) was published in the autumn of 2000. *The NHS Cancer Plan* was an ambitious document setting out a strategy to integrate the prevention, screening, diagnosis, treatment and ongoing care for individuals affected by cancer. It also acknowledged that, to achieve its aims, significant investment was required, not only in the provision of new and replacement equipment, but also in specialist and improved levels of staffing, information systems and drugs. At the heart of the plan was the patient. To ensure that health professionals took into account the views of 'users' (patients and carers) of their services, cancer networks were expected to work with their local service users and voluntary groups, to seek their views for the future provision of cancer services. Indeed, evidence of proactive engagement with service users is subject to assessment via external peer review (DoH, 2004).

After the publication of *The NHS Cancer Plan*, there were over 65 000 responses to a national questionnaire, seeking patients' views on the provision of NHS cancer services (DoH, 2002). The respondents to this questionnaire identified that there could be improvement in the provision of information relating to their diagnosis and treatment, as well as in the support and time available from health professionals (DoH, 2002).

Many of the cancer networks are working with the voluntary organization Cancer-VOICES, which is now part of Macmillan Cancer Support (MCS). CancerVOICES is a national project working with individuals affected by cancer, together with other groups involved in providing support for patients and carers. One of the aims of the project is to encourage those who have experience of cancer services to share that experience and influence the future provision of cancer care (CancerVOICES, 2002). Groups, linked to their local cancer network, are actively working with health professionals on a range of projects, including the development of information materials and guidelines, participation in multiprofessional network groups, development of multiprofessional training programmes and so on (CancerVOICES, 2002). These training programmes not only orientate patients/carers to the workings of the health service, but also facilitate the development of a proactive working relationship between carers and health professionals in order to improve the quality of local cancer services by meeting the needs of the local population – one of the aims of the Calman–Hine Report back in 1995 (DoH, 1995).

Successful treatment, ultimately eradicating the patient's disease, depends very much on how early an individual patient presents and is diagnosed. A 'fast-track' referral system has been implemented throughout the country for all patients visiting their general practitioner (GP) with clinical features suggestive of cancer. As a result of this programme, 99% of all patients with a suspected cancer are seen by the appropriate hospital specialist within two weeks of their referral by a GP (DoH, 2000a; Richards, 2006).

No patient should now wait longer than a month (31 days) from diagnosis to treatment, or two months (62 days) from urgent GP referral to treatment (DoH, 2000a; Richards, 2006). The only exceptions to these waiting times will be: (i) a patient whose clinical condition contraindicates commencement of treatment, for example a patient requiring complex surgery who is found to have an unstable heart condition. Obviously the heart condition will need to be stabilized before the patient is assessed fit for surgery; (ii) a patient who, after receiving adequate information, decides that they would like to defer commencement of treatment for personal reasons, for example a family holiday or wedding.

Faster access to diagnosis and treatment has come at a price. Insufficient staff has meant that not only was an investment in the future workforce required in some areas, but also a coordinated approach to services spanning the whole patient pathway, questioning which is the most appropriate group of health professionals to undertake specific tasks/roles. Training of future staff needs to go hand in hand with ongoing career development. This will ensure not only that individual staff members can realize their full potential, but also that patients can benefit from timely and appropriate care from skilled and knowledgeable health professionals. Individual Trusts are working with their local cancer network and workforce development department (WDD) to develop strategies to meet these challenges (DoH, 2000a). By looking at the patient journey and working with health professionals and service users, bottlenecks in the existing system can be identified, together with innovative ways of overcoming them. This not only leads to a speedier journey for the individual patient, but can also increase capacity within the system, with, for example, nurse-led haematuria clinics, radiographer-led radiotherapy planning, nurse-led follow-up clinics and so on (Richards, 2006).

CANCER SERVICES COLLABORATIVE IMPROVEMENT PARTNERSHIP

The Cancer Services Collaborative Improvement Partnership (CSCIP) is part of the DoH. The CSCIP worked very closely with cancer networks in the early years to look at the provision of specific cancer services within an organization, for example breast services, and map the patient journey. These mapping exercises identified where the delays were for the patient. Before the publication of *The NHS Cancer Plan* (DoH, 2000a), nine cancer networks were already participating in CSCIP projects. The results from these early projects clearly highlighted that many of the delays in a patient's treatment were a result of the way the systems were organized for delivery of care. By working with all the staff involved, the systems could be redesigned to expedite patients' journeys, for example by pre-booking patients at the time of referral for diagnostic tests, based on the information contained in their referral letter (DoH, 2000a). Much of the credit for achieving the two week referral target for individuals with suspected cancer, and the 31- and 62-day targets, belongs to the CSCIP, service improvement leads (SILs) and service improvement facilitators (SIFs) based at both network and acute trust levels. These individuals work closely with health professionals at multidisciplinary team (MDT) and Network Site Specific Groups (NSSG) levels, as well as service users (patients and carers), to identify ways to improve the delivery of cancer services. The *National Manual for Cancer Services* (DoH, 2004) requires each NSSG to have a dedicated person responsible for service improvement, and this is assessed as part of the national peer review programme.

THE PATIENT JOURNEY

Most patients will initially consult their GPs as the first stage in their patient journey. If their GP considers that they have clinical features that could be suggestive of an underlying malignancy, they will be referred to an appropriate specialist under the 'rapid access' criteria (DoH, 2000a, 2000b, 2005). However, a percentage of patients may well present as an emergency, for example with an obstructed bowel, or as a result of 'routine' investigations for symptoms not believed to be related to an underlying malignancy. Or they could be referred into the patient journey following attendance/participation in a cancer screening programme, for example breast screening or bowel screening. Whatever route the patient takes, it is essential that once diagnosis is confirmed, the extent (stage) of the cancer is determined so the patient can be advised on what is/are the most appropriate treatment(s) (see Chapter 1).

In accordance with the *Manual of Cancer Services* (DoH, 2004), all patients should have their management discussed at an MDT meeting. To comply with the *Manual of Cancer Services* (DoH, 2004), a breast MDT should consist of the following 'core' members:

- designated breast surgeon
- breast care nurse(s)
- radiologist (imaging specialist)
- histopathologist
- oncologist (clinical or medical).

In addition to the above, the core team should have access to the following individuals, who are known as 'extended team' members (DoH, 2004):

- palliative care team member
- breast radiographer
- psychiatrist or clinical psychologist
- social worker
- plastic/reconstructive surgeon
- clinical geneticist/genetic counsellor
- physiotherapist/lymphoedema specialist.

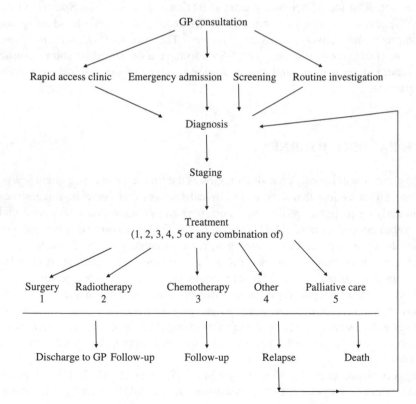

Figure 3.1   The patient pathway (journey).

The discussions at the MDT should ensure that every patient is advised about their most appropriate management by health professionals who are experienced and knowledgeable about their specific cancer. These discussions also ensure that individual patients can benefit from a holistic approach to their care, with support from the site-specific clinical nurse specialist and early onward referral to other members of the team, such as the physiotherapist, palliative care team and so on as appropriate. The patient will also be allocated a 'key worker'. The role of this individual is to act as a point of contact, allowing the patient easy access to members of the multidisciplinary team.

A typical patient journey is depicted in Figure 3.1

THE IMPACT OF RESEARCH ON PATIENT CARE

The NHS Cancer Plan (DoH, 2000a) highlights the importance of research for the detection and treatment of cancer. In particular it highlights the importance of research into the genetic and cellular changes that lead to an individual developing cancer. The *Plan* states:

10.26 The genetic makeup of an individual may determine how effective a particular medicine is and the risk of adverse side effects. Research in this area, known as pharmacogenetics, is accelerating as a result of the Human Genome Project. Genes affecting the metabolism of more than twenty drugs, including anti-cancer agents, have been identified.

10.27 In the future, successful chemotherapy is likely to become increasingly dependent on understanding an individual's genetic background. In partnership with other cancer research funders, we will promote the development of pharmacogenetic studies in the area of cancer chemotherapy.

DoH (2000a, p. 91)

As health-care professionals, we must ensure that every patient has the opportunity to benefit from the latest research and to participate in a clinical trial if it is considered appropriate for his or her individual circumstances. *The NHS Cancer Plan* (DoH, 2000a) states that a review undertaken by the DoH in 1999 considers support for research into cancer a high priority. Thus the National Cancer Research Network (NCRN) was established in April 2001 (*NCRN Newsletter,* November 2001). The aim of the NCRN is to increase the activity and quality of cancer research in the United Kingdom. This has resulted in the establishment of research networks, which are linked closely with the 33 cancer networks. Over a three-year period, from 2001 to 2004, the NCRN aimed to double the number of individual patients recruited into trials. By the summer of 2006 the number of patients recruited into cancer clinical trials had significantly improved throughout the 33 cancer networks in England (Richards, 2006).

Professor Selby (Director of NCRN), writing in the first issue of the *NCRN Newsletter* (November 2001), stated that cancer research would be strengthened by the creation of two additional groups: the National Translational Cancer Research Network (NTRAC) and the National Cancer Research Institute (NCRI). He went on to explain that the NCRI represented the main funders of cancer research, and that NTRAC would be concentrating on the initial development of translational research (see Chapter 11).

CONCLUSION

Although cancer is a common group of diseases, affecting more than a quarter of a million people in the United Kingdom every year, each patient is an individual, and each patient requires information and support pertaining to their individual needs at the various stages of their journey.

Cancer also has an impact on a patient's family and friends. They too require information and support throughout the whole patient journey – and beyond, when treatment options have been exhausted. Patients and carers should be involved in working with health professionals to identify the information and support that are required.

As health professionals, we need to adopt a team approach, ensuring every patient receives the appropriate investigations, treatment and support, accompanied by relevant information, without undue delay. We need to work with our patients and their carers to ensure that they not only receive evidence-based care, but also have the opportunity to participate in clinical trials, if it is appropriate for their individual circumstances. The remaining chapters in this book should help health professionals gain a greater understanding of the research that is taking place to apply the biology of cancer to direct patient care.

Part II   The Science of Cancer

4 The Cell

LOUISE KNIGHT

The human body is made up of about 10 trillion cells and the ability of each of these to produce exact replicas is an essential component of life. In order to begin to understand how things might go wrong and cancer might develop, it is essential to understand normal cellular processes.

WHAT IS A CELL?

The cell is the basic unit of all living matter, whether a single celled bacterium like *Escherichia coli* or a multicelled organism like a human being. Every cell is remarkable; not only do they have the ability to carry out complex tasks, for example uptake of nutrients and conversion to energy, and the ability to replicate, but they also contain all the instructions to carry out these tasks.

Cells are divided into two categories: (1) prokaryotes and (2) eukaryotes:

1. *Prokaryotes* lack a nuclear membrane (the membrane that surrounds the nucleus). The best-known examples of prokaryotic organisms are bacteria. They are composed of a cell envelope, within which the cytoplasmic region is contained. This region contains cytoplasm, which is a fluid made up of about 70% water, the remainder comprising enzymes that the cell has manufactured, amino acids, glucose molecules and adenosine triphosphate (ATP). At the centre of the cell is its DNA, which due to the lack of a nuclear membrane floats within the cytoplasm.
2. *Eukaryotes* contain cell organelles; similarly to organs within the body, each organelle has its own structure and specific function or metabolic process to carry out. Figure 4.1 illustrates some of the organelles that are found within the eukaryotic cell. Among these structures is the nucleus, which is composed of three main parts:

The Biology of Cancer, Second Edition. Edited by J. Gabriel
© 2007 John Wiley & Sons, Ltd.

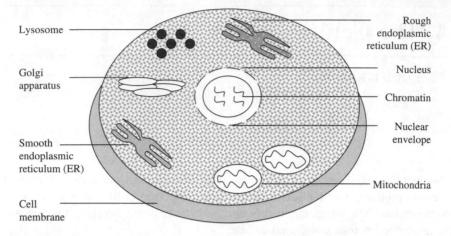

Lysosome

Golgi apparatus

Smooth endoplasmic reticulum (ER)

Cell membrane

Rough endoplasmic reticulum (ER)

Nucleus

Chromatin

Nuclear envelope

Mitochondria

Figure 4.1 A typical eukaryotic cell and some of the components that are found within it.

    i. *Nucleolus.* This is the most prominent part of the nucleus; its function is to produces ribosomes.
   ii. *Nuclear envelope.* This is a double-layered membrane, which protects and separates the nucleus from the cytoplasm and molecules that could cause damage.
  iii. *Chromatin.* This is a DNA/protein complex containing our genes, during replication it condenses into chromosomes.

It is the nucleus that gives the eukaryotye (meaning 'true nucleus') its name. Other important components that are illustrated in the diagram include:

- *Cell membrane.* This comprises a double layer of lipid molecules, which gives the cell support and protection, letting nutrients in and waste molecules out. It is able to alter its shape and receive signals from the outside environment.
- *Mitochondrion.* These are often thought of as the 'power houses' of cells as they are where energy is produced. The mitochondria break down sugar molecules in the presence of oxygen to produce energy in the form of ATP.
- *Rough/Smooth Endoplasmic Reticulum (ER).* These are a series of interconnecting tubular tunnels which are continuous with the outer membrane of the nucleus. The membrane structure of both types is identical, but the rough ER has ribosomes attached to it, as opposed to smooth ER, which does not. The rough ER is involved in protein synthesis, allowing proteins made on the ribosomes to fold into their three-dimensional shape; the smooth ER is the site of steroid production.
- *Lysosomes.* These are spherical bodies containing many digestive enzymes, which are used to break down large molecules.
- *Golgi apparatus.* This is a stack of flattened sacs, associated with the ER. The golgi apparatus modifies proteins and fats, for example adding sugar molecules to form glycoproteins.

(It is important to remember that not all cell organelles have been described within this text. For a detailed description of cell organelles, Alberts *et al.* in *Molecular Biology of the Cell* (2002) is a useful text.)

HOW DOES A CELL DEVELOP AND REPLICATE?

Eukaryotic cells divide to produce two identical daughter cells, each containing exact copies of the DNA from the parent cell; in this way, multicellular organisms are able to replace damaged or worn out cells. The preparation for cell division occurs during interphase, the cell then divides during mitosis, combined these processes form the cell cycle (Figure 4.2).

To the naked eye, interphase appears to be a period of rest for the cell, but in fact much activity is taking place. During this time, RNA is constantly being synthesized, protein is produced and the cell is growing in size. Scientists have determined at a molecular level that the interphase can be divided into the following stages:

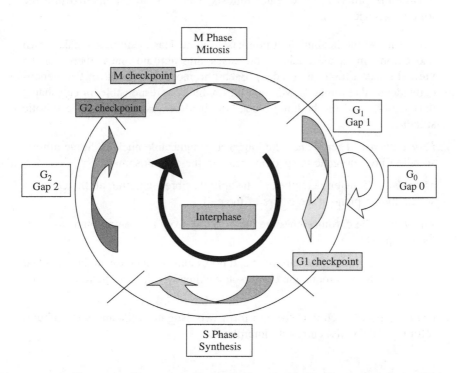

Figure 4.2 Overview of the five stages of normal mammalian cell development. Within each stage there are checkpoints that are regulated by components within the cycle.

Gap 0 (G_0). Cells may leave the cell cycle for a temporary resting period – or more permanently if they have reached the end of their development, for example neurons. Cells in this phase are often termed quiescent and in order to enter back into the cycle they must be stimulated by growth factors, for example platelet-derived growth factor (PDGF). Cells that have permanently stopped dividing due to age or accumulation of cellular damage are termed senescent.

Gap 1 (G_1). Cells increase in size, produce RNA and synthesize protein. There is an important cell cycle control mechanism (checkpoint) activated during this stage (see Section 'Tumour Suppressor Genes') that cells must pass through in order to progress to the S phase.

Synthesis phase (S phase). DNA is replicated during this phase so that the two daughter cells produced following mitosis will contain a copy of the DNA from the parent cell.

Gap 2 (G_2). Cells continue to grow and produce new proteins. At the end of G_2, another important checkpoint is activated (see Section 'Tumour Suppressor Genes').

Now the cell is ready to enter mitosis, which is further divided into the following stages:

Prophase. At the beginning of prophase, the nuclear membrane breaks down and chromatin in the nucleus condenses into chromosomes (these can be viewed under a light microscope). Each chromosome consists of two genetically identical chromatids. Microtubules, which are responsible for cell shape, disassemble, and the building blocks of these are used to form the mitotic spindle.

Prometaphase. There is now no longer a recognizable nucleus. Some mitotic spindle fibres elongate to specific areas on the chromosomes.

Metaphase. Tension is applied to the spindle fibres, aligning all the chromosomes in one plane at the centre of the cell.

Anaphase. The chromosomes are pulled away from the central plane towards the cell poles.

Telophase. Chromosomes arrive at cell poles and decondense, and the nuclear envelope reforms around the clusters at each end of the cell, thereby forming new nuclei.

Cytokinesis. The cell is cleaved to form two daughter cells and microtubules reform for the cells' entry into interphase.

Cells formed by mitosis are said to be diploid because they contain two sets of homologous chromosomes. Another form of cell division to be aware of is meiosis, which occurs only in reproductive cells during the formation of gametes (sex cells).

A cell dividing by meiosis duplicates its DNA as with cells undergoing mitosis, but splits into four new cells instead of two and contains only one copy of each chromosome. These cells are said to be haploid.

(It is often easier to understand the processes described above when you can observe them occurring. A useful web site containing animations and video clips of dividing cells is located at the following address: http://www.cellsalive.com/toc_cellbio.htm.)

HOW IS THE CELL CYCLE CONTROLLED?

Cancer can be described as the uncontrolled proliferation and growth of cells into other tissues. If we can understand the normal mechanisms that control the cell cycle, we can begin to understand how these controls may malfunction and cause cancer to develop. Understanding the cell cycle and its controls also allows the development of specific and targeted therapies to treat the disease.

CYCLINS AND CYCLIN-DEPENDENT KINASES

Many different proteins located within the cytoplasm control the cell cycle; two of the main types are cyclins (the regulatory subunit) and cyclin-dependent kinases (CDKs, the catalytic subunit). A cyclin joins with a CDK to form a complex (cyclin-CDK). If a problem with the cell cycle is detected then activation of the cyclin-CDK complex is not completed. If there are no problems within the cell cycle then formation of the cyclin-CDK is completed. This leads to the activation of a transcription factor by the removal of a transcription factor inhibitor. The transcription factor activates transcription of the genes required for the next stage of the cell cycle, including the cyclin and CDK genes. During the cell cycle, levels of cyclins within the cell will rise and fall but the levels of CDKs will remain fairly constant. Activation of CDKs is a central event in regulating the cell cycle and their activity is therefore regulated at many different levels.

TUMOUR SUPPRESSOR GENES

Tumour suppressor genes prevent excessive growth of a cell; the most well known ones are p53 and the retinoblastoma (Rb) gene.

Retinoblastoma Gene

Retinoblastoma gene is involved in the G_1 checkpoint (Figure 4.2) in the following way. It binds to a family of transcription factors known as the E2F family, thereby repressing their transcription of E2F-responsive genes, such as thymidine kinase (TK), needed for DNA replication, and cyclin E and A, needed for cell cycle progression. Rb is activated when cyclin D forms a complex with CDK4/6 (cyclin

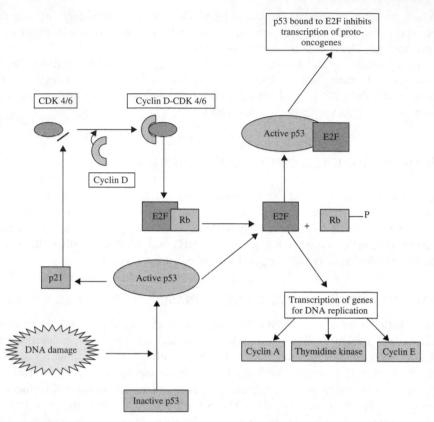

Figure 4.3 If no damage is detected at the G_1 checkpoint, CDK4/6 joins with cyclin D to form a cyclin-CDK complex. This phosphorylates Rb, thereby releasing E2F from its complex and making it active. E2F promotes transcription of E2F responsive genes and hence cell cycle progression. If there is DNA damage, p53 changes from its inactive state to its active state. This triggers transcription of the CDK inhibitor p21, which subsequently blocks the CDK, forming a complex with a cyclin.

D/CDK4/6, hence making it active) this in turn phosphorylates Rb, which allows E2F to be released (Figure 4.3).

p53

The p53 protein is essential for protecting us against cancer. More than half of human cancers have p53 mutations and therefore no functioning p53. p53 works by sensing DNA damage and halting the cell cycle (Figure 4.2). This is essential, because if DNA is damaged but still replicated in S phase, it could eventually manifest in the form of a protein mutation. By halting the cell cycle at the G_1 checkpoint, this can be prevented. So how does this process work? Again, it comes back to the involvement of CDKs. First, in response to a variety of stress signals, for example DNA damage, p53 switches from an inactive state to an active state. It then triggers transcription of the gene for p21, which is a CDK inhibitor. Because active CDKs are needed to progress through the cell cycle, an inactive CDK will cause the cycle to halt.

The p53 protein is also involved at the G_2 checkpoint in cases, for example, where DNA has been synthesized incorrectly. At this checkpoint, p53 binds to E2F (see Section 'Retinoblastoma gene') and prevents it from triggering transcription of proto-oncogenes, for example c-myc and c-fos, which are required for mitosis (Figure 4.3). Proto-oncogenes are important promoters of normal cell growth and division; however, if they become mutated they are known as oncogenes and can have a detrimental effect. A single oncogene cannot cause cancer by itself but it can cause the cell cycle to lose its inhibitory controls, thereby increasing the rate of mitosis. When a cell loses control over mitosis, it can be the beginning of the pathway leading to the development of cancer.

Apoptosis

The main types of DNA repair mechanism operating in mammals are direct reversal, base excision repair, nucleotide excision repair, mismatch repair, non-homologous end joining and recombinational repair; however, these mechanisms are not always successful. If a cell is unable to repair damage to its DNA, the alternative pathway that can be activated is apoptosis, also known as programmed cell death. The signals that induce apoptosis can be extrinsic inducers, for example hormones, or intrinsic inducers, for example viral infection. A cell undergoing apoptosis would exhibit the following specific morphological changes: cell shrinkage, a dense cytoplasm and tightly packed cell organelles, condensation of chromatin, a breakdown of the nuclear envelope, irregular buds known as blebs in the cell membrane, and finally the breaking apart of the cell into several vesicles. Apoptosis therefore involves a series of specific cellular changes that result in the elimination of the cell and hence any mutations within it.

DIFFERENT TYPES OF CELL

The human body is made up of three types of cell: somatic, germ and stem. Somatic cells make up the majority of the body; they have two copies of each chromosome and are therefore diploid. Germ cells give rise to gametes and are constant throughout their generations. Stem cells on the other hand have the ability to divide indefinitely and give rise to specialized cells. For example, blood stem cells can give rise to red blood cells, platelets and white blood cells. Table 4.1 describes some of the different types of tissues within the body and the cells that they are comprised of; most tissues are made up of more than one type of cell.

Table 4.1   Cell and tissue types found within the body and their function

Tissue/Cell type	Function
Epithelia[a]	
Absorptive	These have numerous hairlike structures called microvilli projecting from their surface to increase the surface area for absorption.
Secretory	These are specialized cells that secrete substances onto the surface of the cell sheet. They are often collected together to form a gland that specializes in the secretion of a particular substance. Exocrine glands secrete their products, for example gastric juices, into ducts; endocrine glands secrete into the blood.
Ciliated	These have cilia on their free surface, which beat in synchrony to move substances, for example mucus, over the epithelial sheet.
Connective Tissue	
Fibroblasts	These are located in loose connective tissue and secrete the extra-cellular matrix that fills spaces between organs and tissues.
Osteoblasts	These cells secrete the extracellular matrix in which crystals of calcium phosphate are later deposited to form bone.
Adipose	These are among the largest in the body and produce and store fat. A large lipid droplet within the cell squeezes the nucleus and cytoplasm.
Nervous Tissue	
Neurons	These are specialized cells for communication. The brain and spinal cord are comprised of a network of neurons.
Glial	These are cells that support neurons.
Schwann/ Oligodendrocytes	These wrap around the axon, forming a multilayered membrane sheath. The axon is the structure that conducts electrical signals away from the neuron.
Muscle Tissue	
Skeletal	These are large multinucleated cells that form muscle fibres. Skeletal muscle moves joints by its strong rapid contraction.
Smooth	Composed of thin elongated cells containing one nucleus each. Found in the digestive tract, bladder, arteries and veins.
Cardiac	An intermediate of the previous two types. Cardiac muscle produces the heart beat. Cells are linked by electrically conducting junctions.
Blood	
Erythrocytes (Red blood cells)	These are very small cells, usually with no nucleus or internal membrane. Full of oxygen-binding protein haemoglobin.
Lymphocytes (White blood cells)	These cells protect against infections. They are further sub-divided into lymphocytes, macrophages and neutrophils.
Sensory	
Hair	Sensory cells are some of the most highly specialized cells within the vertebrate body. Hair cells of the inner ear are primary detectors of sound.
Rod	These are found in the retina of the eye and are specialized to respond to light.

[a]Epithelial cells form cell sheets called epithelia. These line the inner and outer surfaces of the body.

WHAT HAPPENS WHEN THE CELL UNDERGOES MALIGNANT CHANGES?

Over the years it has been suggested that the development of cancer is a multi-step process, each step reflecting a genetic change that transforms a normal cell into a malignant cell. A review by Hanahan and Weinberg (2000) summarized these changes as six essential alterations to cell physiology that collectively dictate malignant growth. The alterations are as follows:

Self-sufficiency in growth signals. Normal cells require growth signals to proliferate. Many cancer cells acquire the ability to produce their own growth signals, that is they can synthesize growth factors, to which they also respond. The cells begin to operate as an independent entity as opposed to functioning as part of a larger organism. An example of this is the ability of glioblastomas to produce PDGF (Hermansson *et al.*, 1988).

Insensitivity to inhibitory (antigrowth) signals. Cells monitor their external environment and decide whether to proliferate or not. Many anti-proliferative signals function via the Rb protein (see Section 'Tumour Suppressor Genes'), therefore if this is disrupted, control of the cell cycle is lost and cells will proliferate. This is demonstrated in retinoblastoma cancer, where deletion or mutation of the Rb gene causes tumour growth in one or both eyes in early childhood.

Evasion of apoptosis. Research over the past decade has determined that the apoptotic programme is present in nearly all cells in the body in a latent form. It seems that resistance towards it is a characteristic of most and perhaps all cancers. One way in which apoptosis might be avoided is the loss or mutation of p53, which acts as a proapoptotic regulator by sensing DNA damage.

Limitless replicative potential. Research involving cells in culture has suggested that normal cells can only undergo 60−70 replications, after which time they stop growing and die. Cancer cells however have acquired the capability of endlessly replicating, in many cases due to an enzyme known as telomerase. At the end of every chromosome is a region known as the telomere, which is composed of several thousand repeats of base pairs. During each normal cell replication the telomeres shorten until they can no longer protect the chromosomal DNA, and subsequently the cell dies. However, if telomerase is up-regulated the telomeres will be maintained above a critical length, making the cells immortal.

Sustained angiogenesis. Angiogenesis is the formation of new blood vessels, which is an essential process that must be sustained if the cells in the tumour mass are to be supplied with oxygen and nutrients. It seems that tumours are able to shift the balance of angiogenesis inducers and inhibitors by altering gene expression and, for example, increasing VEGF expression (Hanahan and Folkman, 1996), thereby sustaining angiogenesis.

Tissue invasion and metastasis. The majority of cancer deaths are caused by metastasis of the primary tumour mass to other sites of the body. This begins with the rearrangement of the cells' cytoskeletons, which allows them to attach to other cells and move over or around them. Once they hit a blockage, for example the basal lamina, the cancer cells secrete enzymes to break it down. Included in these enzymes are matrix metalloproteins (MMP), which act as 'molecular scissors' and cut through proteins that might hinder the passage of the cancer cells. Once through the basal lamina, the cells can move into the bloodstream and circulate throughout the body until they find a suitable site to settle on and regrow. A commonly observed alteration that leads to metastasis involves the cell-to-cell interaction molecule E-cadherin. Coupling of this molecule between cells results in transmission of antigrowth signals, acting as a suppressor of invasion and metastasis. It appears that E-cadherin function is lost in the majority of epithelial cancers due to gene mutations.

HOW MAY A PARTICULAR MALIGNANT CONDITION PRESENT?

Different conditions may present themselves in various ways and the earlier the condition is recognized, the better the chance of cure.

COLORECTAL CANCER

Symptoms may include blood or mucus in the faeces; changes in bowel habits (diarrhoea, constipation or both), anything abnormal or that lasts for more than two weeks; the feeling of needing to go to the toilet even if the bowels have just been emptied; pain or discomfort in the abdominal area; a lump in the abdomen; extreme tiredness, which might be due to bleeding. These symptoms may well be present for other reasons, the most common cause of bleeding being haemorrhoids, for example. However, it is important that anyone experiencing these symptoms should see their doctor (Cancer Research UK web site, 2002).

BREAST CANCER

It is important that women know what is normal for them personally and be aware of the following signs: lumps or thickening in the breast or armpit area; changes in the skin in these areas, for example dimpling, redness or puckering; changes in the nipple, for example a change in the direction or an unusual discharge, and also changes around the nipple, for example an unusual rash or sore area; changes to the shape and size of the breast and unusual pain or discomfort, although pain unaccompanied by any other symptoms is unlikely to be due to cancer. These symptoms may be explained by other causes but should still be reported to the doctor (Cancer Research UK web site, 2002).

LUNG CANCER

Symptoms for this disease may not be experienced in the early stages of development and when symptoms do occur they are usually a result of the cancer growing and causing pressure or pain. For example: a persistent cough; wheezing and shortness of breath; blood in the phlegm; recurrent chest infections; chest, shoulder or back pain not related to coughing; a husky voice; unexplained weight loss; fatigue; loss of appetite; unsteady walking; occasional memory lapses; bone fractures not due to an injury (Cancer Research UK web site, 2002).

MELANOMA SKIN CANCER

Small basal cell and squamous cell carcinomas are fairly straightforward to treat and can usually be surgically removed under local anaesthetic. Any pigmented lesion or mole that changes in appearance should be viewed as suspicious and medical attention should be sought. Signs can include a mole that is getting bigger; a change in the shape of the mole, particularly an irregular edge; a mole that is itching, bleeding or has become inflamed or crusty; a change in colour, especially multi-shaded (research has shown that moles with three or more shades of brown or black are particularly likely to be a melanoma) (Cancer Research UK web site,2002).

CONCLUSION

Knowledge of the 'normal' cellular process will help us to understand how things go wrong and to discover ways of preventing/reversing these changes. Cytotoxic chemotherapy and radiotherapy are two approaches that have been used to interfere with the cell cycle and kill malignant cells, but our greater understanding of the cell is leading to other approaches, and these will be discussed further in the next chapter.

5 Cytotoxic Chemotherapy

DEBBIE WRIGHT

[Medicine is] a collection of uncertain prescriptions the results of which, taken collectively, are more fatal than useful to mankind.

Napoleon Bonaparte (1769—1821)

In 1994 the World Health Organization (WHO) stated that just 24 drugs could be considered essential for the rational management of malignant disease. Despite this, the *British National Formulary* 52 lists over 50 cytotoxic agents available for prescription in the United Kingdom. There is little doubt that some of these represent major advances in the fight against cancer but for others the risk:benefit ratio is less clear. Such controversies are not new and arguments have raged over the years concerning the place of chemotherapy in the treatment of neoplastic disease (Bailar and Gornik, 1997; Cunningham, 1995; Kramer and Klausner, 1997; Mead, 1995). In recent times this difficult area has become further complicated by the development of pharmacoeconomics as a science and the growing importance of cost-effectiveness when deciding where resources are best used (Grusenmeyer and Wong, 2007).

This increasing emphasis on the value for money of health interventions, and in particular medicines, is exemplified by the development of the National Institute for Health and Clinical Excellence (formally the National Institute for Clinical Excellence) and its Scottish counterpart, the Scottish Medicines Consortium (SMC). These government funded agencies are tasked to develop guidance on the availability of new and existing drugs and treatments in the National Health Service (NHS). Both clinical and economic evidence is taken into account during the appraisal process. Where the economic case has not been proven, negative decisions have resulted (SMC, 2006). However, as with any evaluation, the interpretation of the data can lead to conflicting as well as harmonious decisions (NICE, 2006, 2007; SMC, 2005).

It is becoming increasingly important to be able to target treatment to those who will benefit most. To achieve this goal, it is necessary to have a thorough understanding of the molecular process involved in the development of cancer, in addition to the pharmacology of the agents in use. The majority of chemotherapy agents

The Biology of Cancer, Second Edition. Edited by J. Gabriel
© 2007 John Wiley & Sons, Ltd.

introduced in the last half of the twentieth century were non-specific, affecting dividing cells with little discrimination (see Chapter 4). This meant that they were destructive not only to cancer cells but also to healthy, rapidly dividing tissues such as the hair follicles and the gastric epithelium, which accounts for many of the adverse effects noted with these agents, such as hair loss and mucositis. An understanding of the molecular biology of cancer, the interactions between malignant cells and their environment, is the first step in designing effective new agents. This approach should improve outcomes and minimize side effects while permitting efficient use of resources.

It has been proposed that an understanding of the actions of anticancer drugs on the cell cycle may provide some insight into which drugs are likely to be of benefit in combination or for specific tumour types. Combination therapy is a common approach that permits enhanced efficacy whilst minimizing toxicity. This holds true where agents with differing pharmacology and adverse effect profiles are prescribed together. It is therefore necessary to understand how current agents work and the cellular processes at play in malignant disease.

MECHANISM OF ACTION OF CHEMOTHERAPY

ALKYLATING AGENTS

The alkylating agents are amongst the oldest anticancer agents still in use today. They were initially investigated as therapeutic agents after it was noted during the First World War that troops exposed to nitrogen mustard 'nerve gas' subsequently developed bone marrow suppression (Hirsch, 2006).

Their name reflects their mechanism of action. These agents add alkyl groups to other molecules, of most relevance to DNA (Hall and Tilby, 1992). They have a threefold effect which accounts for their anticancer properties:

1. They form cross links between base pairs in the DNA double helix, stopping it from uncoiling and separating so replication cannot proceed. This mainly happens with guanine, although adenine and cytosine may also be affected.
2. Alkyl groups attach to DNA bases, which results in fragmentation of the DNA by repair enzymes.
3. Attachment of alkyl groups to DNA base pairs results in mismatched pairing of the nucleotides, leading in turn to DNA mutations.

Not surprisingly, alkylating agents are cell cycle non-specific. The S phase is where the effects largely manifest, resulting in a block at G2 (Rang *et al.*, 2003).

Uses

The non-specific action of alkylating agents means they are effective in a wide range of tumour types, including those affecting the brain, breast, lymphomas, leukaemias and sarcomas, among others (Ardeshna *et al.*, 2003; Bonnadonna *et al.*, 1976; Chang *et al.*, 2004; van Oosterom *et al.*, 2002).

Examples. Busulfan, carmustine, chlorambucil, cyclophosphamide, dacarbazine, estramustine, ifosfamide, lomustine, melphalan, temozolamide, thiotepa, treosulfan.

CYTOTOXIC ANTIBIOTICS AND AMSACRINE

A number of agents in this class are derived from natural sources such as bacteria (Takeuchi, 1995). They work by:

- intercalation with DNA
- DNA strand breakage
- inhibition of topoisomerase II, an enzyme responsible for uncoiling and repairing damaged DNA.

Some may also affect RNA polymerase activity, stopping transcription, or regulate gene expression and be involved in the production of free radical damage to DNA. It is thought that others may act by inhibiting B cell, T cell and macrophage proliferation, and by impairing antigen presentation and secretion of interferon gamma, TNFα and interleukin II (Gamba-Vitalo *et al.*, 1987).

Amsacrine, while not strictly a cytotoxic antibiotic, has a similar mechanism of action. It promotes double strand breaks in DNA by intercalation, mainly through AT pairs. It also affects topoisomerase II, so it is most effective in the S phase when this enzyme is at the height of its activity (Finlay *et al.*, 1999).

Bleomycin differs from the other members of this class in that it chelates ferrous iron and interacts with oxygen to generate superoxide and/or hydroxyl free radicals. These in turn degrade preformed DNA. Bleomycin has its major effect in the G_2 and M phases of cell division, although it also affects non-dividing cells — that is, G_0 (Hecht, 2000).

As with the alkylating agents, the cytotoxic antibiotics are non-cell-phase specific.

Uses

These agents may be used in treating germ cell, melanoma, breast, colorectal, myeloma and prostate cancers (Berry *et al.*, 2002; Chester *et al.*, 2000; Coskun *et al.*, 2003; Samson *et al.*, 1989).

Examples. Bleomycin, dactinomycin, daunorubicin, doxorubicin, epirubicin, idarubicin, mitomycin, mitoxantrone.

ANTI-METABOLITES

The term anti-metabolite is used to cover a number of cytotoxic agents that act by masquerading as purines or pyrimidines, the building blocks of DNA. The means by which they do this vary from agent to agent. For example, methotrexate interferes with the action of the enzyme dihydrofolate reductase. Dihydrofolate reductase is necessary for the conversion of folates to tetrahydrofolate, an essential agent for the synthesis of thymidylate, hence DNA and purines (Kamen, 1997). Fluorouracil, in contrast, is an analogue of uracil which interferes with the same pathway, but this time at the level of the enzyme thymidylate synthetase (Danenberg, Malli and Swenson, 1999). The end result is the same; inhibition of DNA synthesis but not RNA or protein synthesis. Other agents, such as cytarabine and fludarabine, are analogues of naturally occurring nucleosides, such as 2-deoxycytadine and purine, respectively. Despite the difference, both agents ultimately promote cell death by preventing the action of DNA polymerase (Gandhi and Plunkett, 1994). This action on DNA replication means that the cytotoxic antibiotics are cell cycle specific, acting principally during the S phase of cell division.

Uses

This class of drug is active against a number of tumours, including bladder, breast, colorectal and lung cancer, as well as leukaemias and lymphomas (van Cutsem *et al.*, 2001; Klasa *et al.*, 2002; Reichardt *et al.*, 2003; Vogelzang *et al.*, 2003; Hellenic Co-operative Group, 2004).

Examples. Capecitabine, cladribine, cytarabine, fludarabine, fluorouracil, gemcitabine, mercaptopurine, methotrexate, pemetrexed, raltitrexed, tegafur with uracil, tioguanine.

VINCA ALKALOIDS AND ETOPOSIDE

The vinca alkaloids were originally derived from the periwinkle plant *Catharanthus roseus*. Their activity results from an ability to bind to microtubular proteins present in the mitotic spindle, leading in turn to crystallization of the microtubule and mitotic arrest. Although interference with mitosis is the principal action of the vinca alkaloids, they may also produce their cytotoxic effects by numerous secondary actions (Dumontet and Sikic, 1999; Jordan and Wilson, 2004; Nagle, Hur and Gray, 2006).

In contrast, etoposide, a derivative of the mandrake plant, has no action on the mitotic spindle. Instead its pharmacology is more in line with that of doxorubicin, an inhibition of DNA topoisomerase II preventing DNA synthesis. As with the vinca alkaloids, etoposide is cell cycle dependent and phase specific, working in the S and G_2 phases of cell division (Hartman and Lipp, 2006).

Uses

The vinca alkaloids are used in a variety of tumours, including brain and breast tumours, lymphomas and lung cancer (Le Chevalier *et al.*, 1994; Weber *et al.*, 1995; Burton *et al.*, 2006). Etoposide is also active against a range of malignant processes, such as germ cell malignancies, lung cancer and lymphomas (Pronzato *et al.*, 1994; De Witt *et al.*, 2001).

Examples. Etoposide, vinblastine, vincristine, vindesine, vinorelbine.

PLATINUM COMPOUNDS

Cisplatin was the first of this class to be synthesized, as long ago as 1845. Despite this, its potential as an antitumour agent was not recognized until the 1960s, and it was a decade after that before the initial clinical trials took place and the drug was introduced into clinical practice (Lippert, 1999). The action of the platinum compounds is analogous to that of the alkylating agents. On entering the cell they form a reactive complex that interacts with DNA and forms intrastrand cross links between adjacent guanine molecules (Muggia and Fojo, 2004).

These agents are considered to be non-cell-cycle specific.

Uses

The platinum agents have achieved widespread use in the treatment of bladder cancer, colorectal cancer, upper gastrointestinal disease, germ cell tumours, head and neck malignancies, lung cancer and ovarian cancer (Bellmut *et al.*, 1997; Marth *et al.*, 1998; De Witt *et al.*, 2001; White *et al.*, 2001).

Examples. Carboplatin, cisplatin, oxaliplatin.

TAXANES

Derivatives of the American yew tree, the taxanes are similar to those other plant based molecules, the vinca alkaloids, in that they act on microtubules. However, the process by which this occurs is subtly different. The taxanes stabilize the structure of the microtubules by binding to tubulin, an essential building block of the microtubules. The microtubule–taxane complex is unable to disassemble, a process that is necessary for vital interphase and mitotic cellular functions. The taxanes may also induce programmed cell death by binding to Bcl-2, an apoptosis stopping protein, thus arresting its function. The taxanes act in the G_2 and M phases of the cell cycle (Dumontet and Sikic, 1999; Jordan and Wilson, 2004).

Uses

Breast cancer, germ cell tumours, head and neck malignancies, lung and ovarian cancer can all be treated by utilizing a taxane-based regimen (Motzer, Sheinfeld and Mazumdar, 2000; O'Shaughnessy *et al.*, 2002; Rosenberg *et al.*, 2002; Schiller *et al.*, 2002; Hitt *et al.*, 2005).

Examples. Docetaxel, paclitaxel.

CAMPTOTHECINS

The camptothecins are one of the several cytotoxic agents derived from a natural plant source; in this instance, the *Camptotheca accuminata* tree. They interfere with the action of topoisomerase I, an enzyme that is necessary for DNA replication to occur. Topoisomerase I relieves the torsional strain on DNA by inducing reversible single strand breaks. The camptothecins are S phase specific (Hartman and Lipp, 2006).

Uses

The camptothecins are principally used in the treatment of colorectal, lung and ovarian cancer (Scheithauer *et al.*, 2003; Ten Bokkel Huinink *et al.*, 2004).

Examples. Irinotecan, topotecan.

NON-CYTOTOXIC CANCER AGENTS

In the early twenty-first century there has been a rapid growth in the development of agents active in the treatment of various malignancies that are not, by definition, traditional cytotoxics, that is, that do not directly interfere with DNA. Instead, many affect cellular signalling pathways or are based on antibody technology.

Tyrosine Kinase Inhibitors

The tyrosine kinases are a diverse group of enzymes that are involved in a variety of cellular processes. Receptors for many signalling proteins, such as vascular endothelial growth factor, sit on the surface of cells, including those that are malignant. Once receptor activation has occurred, a tyrosine kinase enzyme within the cell triggers a chemical signal that eventually leads to, for example, cell growth and division (Faivre *et al.*, 2006).

There are drugs available that either inhibit activation of the enzyme by binding to the cell surface receptor or else directly inhibit the enzyme itself. Some are multi-targeted and able to prevent the action of a number of signalling proteins at once (Faivre *et al.*, 2006).

Uses

The tyrosine kinase inhibitors are an emerging group of drugs that so far have found applications in the treatment of leukemias, lung cancer, renal cell disease and sarcomas.

Examples. Erlotinib, imatinib, sorafinib, sunitinib.

PROTEOSOME INHIBITORS

Tyrosine kinases are not the only enzymes involved in signalling processes. Proteosomes are another example and are found in cells throughout the body. Again their actions are far reaching and they have an important role in controlling cell function and growth. The first proteosome inhibitor to be made commercially available was bortezomib, a reversible inhibitor of the 26S proteosome. This particular proteosome degrades various proteins that are critical to cancer cell survival, such as cyclins, among others. The cell becomes sensitized to apoptosis. In addition, bortezomib may enhance the sensitivity of cells to more traditional cancer drugs (Nencioni *et al.*, 2007).

Uses

At present, bortezomib is indicated for the treatment of multiple myeloma (Nencioni *et al.*, 2007).

Example. Bortezomib.

MONOCLONAL ANTIBODIES

Monoclonal antibodies are immunoglobulins, produced by cell cultures, that are selected to react with an antigen specifically expressed on a cancer cell, for example HER2 in breast cancer. The antibody attaches to the specific antigen, which in turn activates the host immune system, resulting in tumour cell death by means of complement mediated lysis or attack by killer cells (Tobinai, 2007). Some monoclonals may attach to and subsequently deactivate growth factor receptors on cancer cells, promoting apoptosis. Bevacizumab acts in this way by binding to vascular endothelial growth factor (Shih and Lindley, 2006).

Some antibodies are in clinical use as part of a radioisotope treatment programme (Cheson, 2003).

Uses

The monoclonal antibodies are currently in use for breast and colorectal cancer, head and neck tumours, leukaemias and lymphomas (Cheson, 2003; Shih and Lindley, 2006, Smith *et al.*, 2007; Tobinai, 2007).

Examples. Alemtuzumab, bevacizumab, cetuximab, gemtuzumab, ibritumomab tiuxetan, rituximab, trastuzumab.

OTHERS

There are a number of other cytotoxic agents that cannot be classified easily into the above categories, for example procarbazine. Procarbazine undergoes transformation to active metabolites that interfere with mitosis at interphase, hence inhibiting the production of both DNA and RNA (Newell *et al.*, 1987).

Bexarotene is a retinoid that selectively activates retinoid X receptors. Once activated, these receptors function as transcription factors, regulating the expression of genes controlling cellular differentiation and proliferation (Farol and Hymes, 2004).

Hydroxycarbamide is a urea analogue that interferes with the conversion of ribonucleotides to deoxyribonucleotides by preventing the action of ribonucleotide reductase (Hong and Erusalimsky, 2002).

Uses

The diversity of these agents means they are active across a range of malignant diseases from brain tumours to leukaemias, cutaneous lymphomas and myelomas (Cairncross *et al.*, 2006, Heald *et al.*, 2003).

Examples. Amsacrine, arsenic trioxide, bexarotene, crisantaspase, hydroxycarbamide, pentostatin, procarbazine, tretinoin.

NON-CYTOTOXIC THERAPY

In addition to the traditional cytotoxic agents and those that affect signalling pathways, there a number of other agents commonly used in cancer that do not affect the cell cycle as such. Included under this umbrella are the hormone antagonists used in breast and prostate cancer; mitotane, which prevents the synthesis of adrenal hormones; thalidomide for myeloma; and the cytokines, such as interferon, commonly prescribed for renal cell cancer and melanoma (Ciberra *et al.*, 2006; Howell *et al.*, 2005; Motzer *et al.*, 2007; SMC, 2006).

Uses

Hormone sensitive tumours such as breast, prostate and adrenal tumours, myeloma and renal cell carcinoma (Ciberra *et al.*, 2006; Howell *et al.*, 2005; Motzer *et al.*, 2007; SMC, 2006).

Examples. Anastrozole, bicalutamide, buserelin, cyproterone, exemestane, flutamide, fulvestrant, goserelin, letrozole, leuprorelin, mitotane, tamoxifen, trilostane, toremifene, triptorelin, thalidomide.

THE FUTURE

The treatment of cancer remains one of the most active areas of research in medicine, in terms of both drugs and the physiological pathways responsible for the development of malignancies.

In addition to the processes already described, there are a number of other pathways that are potential targets for novel anticancer agents. The Ras protein regulates signalling pathways. Farnesyl protein transferases are necessary for the action of Ras, so inhibitors of these enzymes are under investigation (Zangani, 2006).

The ability of tumour cells to grow and divide is partly dependent on their ability to produce metalloproteinases and angiogenesis factors, both of which are known to facilitate tumour growth, the invasion of normal tissues and metastasis. It is not surprising that these pathways are also being targeted in the development of new anticancer therapies (Zucker *et al.*, 2000).

Antisense oligonucleotides are further compounds currently in clinical development. These are essentially synthetic sequences of single stranded DNA which are complementary to specific regions of mRNA that inhibit gene expression (Wacheck and Zangemeister-Wittke, 2006).

CONCLUSION

Cancer is a complex disease that is heterogeneous in nature. As our understanding of the processes involved in the transformation of healthy to malignant cells grows, so too will the potential sites for new targeted agents. It remains an exciting time for the development of anticancer drugs.

6 What Are DNA and RNA?

SCOTT C. EDMUNDS

It is now common knowledge that DNA (deoxyribonucleic acid) is the carrier of genetic information in all living cells (Watson and Crick, 1953). It has, however, been a long, slow process to explain how this relatively simple-structured molecule carries all that genetic information and enables the existence of all of the richly varied life on our planet. The DNA molecule stores information coding for the instructions needed to make a living organism. It does this in a similar way to the digital coding that makes up a computer program. But where computer memory uses a binary system of ones and zeroes (e.g. 1101 10111010010110), the genetic code uses repeating subunits of the DNA molecule (e.g. TAG, GAT, TAC CAT). This molecule has to be able to perform many complicated tasks, such as replicating itself perfectly. It also needs to be able to translate its genetic message into an intermediate message molecule (now known to be RNA) that can travel to the protein-producing machinery of the cell, and then make all of the tens of thousands of different proteins that make up an organism (Figure 6.1).

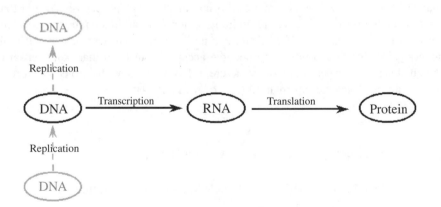

Figure 6.1 DNA makes RNA makes protein – the fundamental dogma of molecular biology.

The Biology of Cancer, Second Edition. Edited by J. Gabriel
© 2007 John Wiley & Sons, Ltd.

BACKGROUND

Looking at the resemblances between parent and child, it is obvious that physical traits are inherited. The ancient Greeks were the first to formulate a scientific theory for how this could work – the theory of 'pangenesis', where representative particles from all over the body pass as hereditary material through the semen. This theory held sway until the eighteenth and nineteenth centuries. It was not until the 1860s that Gregor Mendel, a Czech monk who did breeding experiments with common garden peas, first reported the basic laws of genetic inheritance. From these experiments, Mendel hypothesized that phenotypical (physical) traits are the result of the interaction of 'discrete particles' (now called 'genes') provided by both parents and passed to their offspring (Allen, 2003).

Mendel's theories were almost universally ignored during his lifetime, but were rediscovered in 1900, many years after his death. The discovery of chromosomes at around that time – and their similarity in behaviour to Mendel's 'discrete particles'– led to Walter Sutton's 'chromosomal theory of inheritance' in 1903. Although scientists were convinced that the hereditary material resided in these chromosomes, they were puzzled over what substance carried this information. From chemical analysis it was discovered that the chromosomes were made of both DNA and protein. Initially it was not thought that DNA could carry the genetic code; it seemed too simple a molecule – linear and made up of monotonous repeating sequences of four subunits. Proteins are far more complicated molecules, with up to 20 different subunits, and complicated three-dimensional branched and globular structures.

It was not until the 1940s and 1950s that scientists started to accept evidence that DNA was the carrier of genetic information. In 1944, Avery discovered that bacteria called pneumococci could be transformed from an innocuous to a virulent form by the addition of purified DNA extract from other virulent bacteria. It took several years for these findings to become accepted, but from that point onwards the challenge was to determine the structure of DNA, and how the molecule worked as the carrier of genetic information (Avery *et al.,* 1944).

DETERMINING THE STRUCTURE OF DNA

DNA was found to be a long chain of nucleotides consisting of three parts:

1. deoxyribose, a pentose (five-carbon) sugar
2. phosphoric acid
3. one of four organic (nitrogenous) bases. These organic bases are either the purines adenine (A) and guanine (G) or the pyrimidines cytosine (C) and thymine (T) (Voet and Voet, 1995).

How these four repeating subunits come together to form the genetic code now had to be explained. A major clue was discovered by Erwin Chargaff (Chargaff *et al.*, 1951), who noted that, despite the seemingly large variation in the composition of these four bases from organism to organism, DNA always has an equal number of adenine and thymine residues (A = T) and of guanine and cytosine bases (G = C). This relationship is now known as 'Chargaff's rule'. The other crucial piece of evidence came from X-ray diffraction photography experiments on the DNA molecule, carried out by Maurice Wilkins and Rosalind Franklin (Wilkins, Stokes and Wilson, 1953) at King's College in London, which showed that DNA must be a helical molecule.

Using these findings, two young scientists at Cambridge University, James Watson and Francis Crick, finally determined the structure of DNA − giving rise to the so-called 'Watson−Crick' model. This discovery and its publication in the journal *Nature* in 1953 were said by many to mark the birth of molecular biology (Watson and Crick, 1953). Crick, Watson and Wilkins won the Nobel Prize for Chemistry in 1964 (by this time Rosalind Franklin had died), and the way was clear for tremendous strides in our understanding of DNA − arguably the central molecule of life. In addition to providing the structure of this molecule, the Watson−Crick model also suggests the molecular mechanism for heredity (Watson and Crick, 1953).

THE PRIMARY STRUCTURE OF DNA

Individual nucleotides form a polynucleotide linear polymer, where each mononucleotide monomer unit is linked by chemical bonds known as phosphodiester bridges. These bonds link the 3′-carbon in the ribose of one deoxynucleotide to the 5′-carbon in the ribose of the adjacent deoxynucleotide (for an overview, see Voet and Voet, 1995) (Figure 6.2).

The genome of all living cells is composed of double-stranded DNA containing two anti-parallel polynucleotide chains. This is because the organic bases project into the centre of the molecule (with the phosphate and ribose groups acting as a backbone on the outside) and form base-pairs joined by non-covalent hydrogen bonds. Adenine links to thymine only via two hydrogen bonds, and guanidine links to cytosine via three hydrogen bonds. This makes two anti-parallel strands with their 5′ to 3′ directions being in opposite directions to each other. This specificity of base-pairing thus allows precise duplication of DNA, while holding the two strands tightly together. The geometry of these Watson−Crick base-pairs makes these two DNA strands wrap around together, forming a double helix. In double-stranded DNA there is one turn of the helix every 3.4 nm (Watson and Crick, 1953).

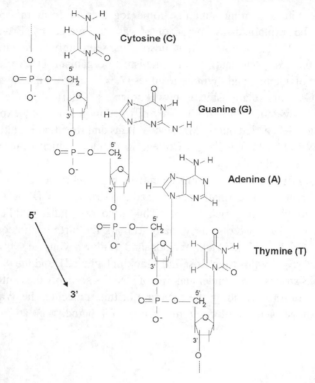

Figure 6.2 The structure of the DNA molecule.

SOME FACTS

The bacterium *Escherichia coli* has a single circular DNA molecule of 4.6 million base-pairs, making the total length of this single DNA molecule around 1.4 mm. In humans there are around 3 billion letters in the DNA code. In a single diploid cell, if fully extended, the DNA would have a length of almost 2 m. If all the DNA of the roughly 50 trillion cells in the human body were unwrapped and placed end to end, it would reach from the earth to the moon roughly 100 000 times! (Kothari and Mehta, 2002).

Fortunately, DNA in the human cell is not unwound, because it needs to be contained within a nucleus only 10 μm in diameter. DNA is wrapped up with proteins called histones. The DNA molecule wraps around several types of histone protein, collected into a structure known as a nucleosome. These nucleosomes, with DNA wrapped around, fold up further, forming the chromosomes. How tightly folded this DNA is varies according to what the DNA is encoding, and what process it is undergoing at a particular time (Kornberg and Lorch, 1999).

The genetic information needs to be able to carry out three functions. A gene needs to replicate itself, making a perfect copy every time the cell divides, a process known as replication. The replicated gene must be able to transfer its genetic message to

RNA molecules in order to make a protein, a process known as transcription. Using this message, the protein has to be manufactured from individual amino acid units, a process known as translation (Voet and Voet, 1995).

REPLICATION

The specific Watson–Crick base-pairing and double helical structure of the DNA molecule has made it quite easy to deduce the copying mechanism for the genetic material. The two parent strands of the double helix are unwound, with each strand acting as a template for the synthesis of a complementary daughter strand. Free nucleotides floating in the nucleoplasm have a free triphosphate group on the 5′-carbon atom of the sugar, and this bonds with a hydroxyl group on the template. This means that the chain can grow only in a 5′ to 3′ direction. This process is catalysed by the enzyme DNA polymerase. As the DNA chains can grow only in a 5′ to 3′ direction, one of the strands is replicated in a series of short discontinuous pieces as the parental helix unwinds. These short fragments are subsequently joined up by another enzyme, known as DNA ligase. The parental duplex is thus replicated to form two daughter duplexes, each consisting of one parental strand and one newly synthesized daughter strand (Figure 6.3) (Lewin, 2004).

TRANSCRIPTION

The genetic information held in the DNA has to direct the production of all of the proteins that build up in a cell, and then in a whole organism. As proteins are produced in the cytoplasm, and the DNA is held in the nucleus, an intermediary 'transcript' molecule has to pass this information to the protein-making machinery. This intermediary molecule is another nucleic acid very similar to DNA, known as ribonucleic acid or RNA. RNA differs in structure from DNA in that its pentose sugar is a ribose rather than deoxyribose, and the organic base thymine is replaced by a different pyrimidine called uracil. Uracil (U) acts as the complementary base to adenine, and all of the bases in RNA can bind and form a complementary strand to a DNA template. This allows a RNA copy of the genetic message to be produced, in a fundamentally similar way to DNA replication, except that only one of the DNA strands is ever copied. This makes RNA a single-stranded molecule (Voet and Voet, 1995).

There are three major classes of RNA: messenger RNA (mRNA), ribosomal RNA (rRNA) and transfer RNA (tRNA) (Lewin, 2003). As its name suggests,

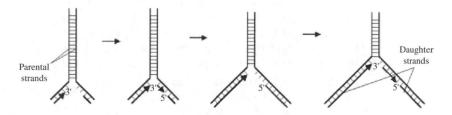

Figure 6.3 DNA replication.

mRNA is the carrier of the genetic message; the other RNAs (tRNA and rRNA) are structural RNAs that are part of the protein-making machinery. Thousands of different mRNAs can be produced and transported around a single cell, each one transcribed from different genes, with each transcript coding for a different protein.

There are 20 amino acids. The four nucleotides that make up the genetic code need to be able to encode the instructions for proteins containing any number of these 20 units, as well as providing at least one code giving instructions for when the protein-making machinery should start or stop. To code for this number of amino acids and start/stop instructions, a language based on nucleotide triplets is used, which is normally represented as groups of three letters, for example TAG.CGE, AGC and so on. There are 64 possible triplets that can be coded for ($4^3 = 64$). Thus, the mRNA sequence is read as a number of triplets, or 'codons', each codon specifying the insertion of a specific amino acid into the growing protein chain. Initiation of translation begins at an initiation codon, AUG, which is also the code for the amino acid methionine. Termination of protein synthesis is coded by one of three different termination codons: UAA, UAG or UGA. As there are 64 possible codons in the genetic code and only 20 different amino acids, the code is said to be degenerate, most amino acids being encoded by more than one codon. Some amino acids, for example alanine, can be encoded by four codons (GCU, GCC, GCA and GCG), whereas others, for example tryptophan, are encoded by only one (UGG) (see Table 6.1) (Lewin, 2003).

The mRNA of eukaryotic organisms is modified in several ways before it can be translated. The mRNA molecule is capped at both ends, possibly to prevent

Table 6.1   The Genetic Code

First Letter	Second Letter				Third Letter
	U	C	A	G	
U	UUU (Phe)	UCU (Ser)	UAU (Tyr)	UGU (Cys)	U
	UUC (Phe)	UCC (Ser)	UAC (Tyr)	UGC (Cys)	C
	UUA (Leu)	UCA (Ser)	UAA (Stop)	UGA (Stop)	A
	UUG (Leu)	UCG (Ser)	UAG (Stop)	UGG (Trp)	G
C	CUU (Leu)	CCU (Pro)	CUA (His)	CGU (Arg)	U
	CUC (Leu)	CCC (pro)	CAC (His)	CGC (Arg)	C
	CUA (Leu)	CCA (Pro)	CAA (Gln)	CGA (Arg)	A
	CUG (Leu)	CCG (Pro)	CAG (Gln)	CGG (Arg)	G
A	AUU (Ile)	ACU (Thr)	AAU (Asn)	AGU (Ser)	U
	AUC (Ile)	ACC (Thr)	AAC (Asn)	AGC (Ser)	C
	AUA (Ile)	ACA (Thr)	AAA (Lys)	AGA (Arg)	A
	AUG (Met)	ACG (Thr)	AAG (Lys)	AGG (Arg)	G
G	GUU (Val)	GCU (Ala)	GAU (Asp)	GGU (Gly)	U
	GUC (Val)	GCC (Ala)	GAC (Asp)	GGC (Gly)	C
	GUA (Val)	GCA (Ala)	GAA (Glu)	GGA (Gly)	A
	GUG (Val)	GCG (Ala)	GAG (Glu)	GGG (Gly)	G

premature degradation and possibly to help guide the molecule to the protein-making machinery. A modified nucleotide base, a methylated guanine residue, caps the 5′ end. The 3′ end is capped by 100–200 adenine residues, and is known as the poly-A tail. Most genes of higher organisms are interrupted by segments of non-coding DNA. These genes are made up of patches of coding (exons) interspersed with non-coding sequence (introns). These introns are removed from the mRNA or spliced before the mRNA leaves the nucleus. This mechanism of rearranging introns and exons gives the organism flexibility in mixing and matching different functional parts of genes to create different splice forms with different functions (Patel and Steitz, 2003).

TRANSLATION

Translation is mRNA-directed biosynthesis of protein. The protein-making machinery produces the specific protein (polypeptide) by a cytoplasmic organelle known as the ribosome. The ribosome is part protein and part structural RNA, known as rRNA. When mRNA binds to the ribosome, translation can start. Each amino acid is carried to the site of protein synthesis by an intermediary molecule known as tRNA. There is a specific tRNA for each amino acid, each one binding to the mRNA triplet that encodes that amino acid. This binding is via an anticodon loop on the tRNA molecule, which contains three nucleotides that base-pair to each mRNA codon. The ribosome provides a site for this binding to occur, starting first with the AUG initiation codon. The ribosome moves along the mRNA molecule in a 5′ to 3′ direction; each amino acid is brought into place by a tRNA molecule and then covalently bonded by enzymes to form a peptide (protein) chain. The ribosome falls off the mRNA chain when it reaches the termination codon, by which time it has produced a complete protein chain (Alberts *et al.*, 2002).

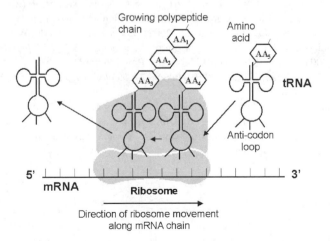

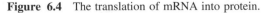

Figure 6.4 The translation of mRNA into protein.

The completed polypeptide chain contains signals that direct post-translational processing and transport to different cellular/extracellular compartments. More than one ribosome can bind to an mRNA molecule at any one time, and the number of ribosomes bound can determine the rate of translation (Figure 6.4) (Alberts *et al.*, 2002).

CONCLUSION

The synthesis of all the body's proteins using the genetic code as a template has to be a very precise process. Protein after protein has to be produced in exactly the same way so that the function is not altered. The genetic code must not alter over generation after generation of cell division in every single cell, and across the trillions of cells that make up the human body. The specificity of the base pairing of the two antiparallel strands is what allows precise duplication of this code. Various enzymes proofread the DNA to make sure that any wrongly incorporated bases are removed. Despite this, errors in DNA replication do occur. If mutations occur inside transcribed parts of the genome, problems may arise. Mutations in the special promoter regions at the beginnings of genes can mean that the protein is not produced at all. Entire genes may be deleted, and mutations inside the exons of genes may produce mutant proteins that may have altered and disrupted function. These altered or missing proteins are implicated in many disorders and diseases, including cancer.

FURTHER SOURCES

Alberts, B., Johnson, A., Lewis, J., Raff, M., Roberts, K. and Walter, P. (2002) *Molecular Biology of the Cell*, 4th edn, Garland: Garland, London and New York.
Berg, J.M., Tymoczko, J.L. and Stryer, L. (2002) *Biochemistry*, 5th edn, W.H. Freeman.
Kuhn, H. and Waser, J. (1994) On the origin of the genetic code. *FEBS Lett*, **352**(3).
Lewin, B. (2004) *Genes VIII*, Oxford University Press, Oxford.
Strachan, T. and Read, A.P. (1999) *Human Molecular Genetics II*, BIOS Scientific Publishers, Oxford.
Voet, D. and Voet, J.G. (1995) *Biochemistry*, John Wiley & Sons.
Watson, J. D. (2004) *DNA: The Secret of Life*, Arrow.
Williams, J.G., Ceccarelli, A. and Spurr, N. (2001) *Genetic Engineering*, 2nd edn (Medical Perspectives Series), Springer.

7 Genetics and Cancer

SCOTT C. EDMUNDS

WHAT ARE GENES?

As mentioned in Chapter 6, DNA is a molecule that contains genetic code, encoding all the proteins that make up an organism. The human genome, the total amount of genetic material of which a human cell is composed, is made up of roughly 20 000–25 000 genes (International Human Genome Sequencing Consortium, 2004); single coding units of DNA that encode for each of the proteins produced by a human. If the genetic code of any gene is altered in any way (e.g. by a mutation) there can be potentially serious consequences for gene expression. This is particularly the case in genes that affect the health and life of the organism directly. If the structure or expression levels are abnormally altered in any of the countless proteins involved in the cellular processes essential for life, this can give rise to life-threatening illnesses, including disorders such as cancer (Hansen and Cavenee, 1988).

MUTATIONS

As most of the human genome is non-coding DNA sequence, called 'junk DNA', most genetic changes are usually harmless. Only about 1.5% of the human genome accounts for the coding sequence, and genes are split into coding and non-coding regions, known as exons (coding) and introns (non-coding), which are spliced together during transcription; therefore only mutations in exonic regions will affect the amino acid composition of a protein (Lewin, 2004). Upstream (the 5′end) of the coding regions of any gene lie non-coding regions essential for gene expression, known as promoter and enhancer elements. These give instructions for where the gene expression machinery should start transcription of the mRNA message, and what levels of transcript should be produced. Any alterations to the genetic coding of these regions can potentially affect the expression of a gene (Lewin, 2004). Any alterations to regions around the splice sites of introns and exons, known as intron–exon junctions, can affect the splicing and exonic structure of a gene (Strachan and Read, 1999).

The nature of the genetic alteration affects the severity of the consequence. Less severe mutations include single-base substitutions. The most common and best

The Biology of Cancer, Second Edition. Edited by J. Gabriel
© 2007 John Wiley & Sons, Ltd.

characterized sources of genetic variation between individuals are these single-base substitutions, which are also known as single-nucleotide polymorphisms (SNPs) (Weiner and Hudson, 2002). Some single-base substitutions have no effect on amino acid composition and are known as 'silent mutations' (Lewin, 2004). More serious alterations to the gene are substitutions amd deletions, with one or more nucleotides inserted or removed. Larger-scale chromosomal abnormalities can also arise, where regions of the chromosome are gained or lost, or entire parts of the chromosome are broken and rejoined to other chromosomes. Mutations in DNA can be produced by errors in DNA replication and repair. The enzymes that control DNA replication are very efficient, and there are many proofreading and repair mechanisms in place to prevent dangerous mutations occurring. As a result of the sheer size of the human genome (3 billion base-pairs), the number of cells in the body and the number of times a cell will divide throughout a human's lifetime, it is no surprise that errors do sometimes occur. Mutations can also be induced by external factors such as mutagenic chemicals and radiation. Mutations occurring in the germ cells (sperm and eggs) can be passed on from generation to generation. Those occurring in single cells, known as somatic changes, are not passed on (Strachan and Read, 1999).

SINGLE-BASE SUBSTITUTIONS

Individual base substitutions are among the most common mutations. As each amino acid is specified by a codon consisting of three bases, if a single base is substituted the altered sequence may code for a different amino acid. It will not necessarily have this effect, however; several codons can code for the same amino acid. As there are two different codons that code for lysine, if the final base-pair of the codon AAA was converted from an A to a G (i.e. AAG) this would be a silent mutation as both AAA and AAG encode for lysine. There are many other examples of this, because most amino acids are encoded by more than one codon (Lewin, 2004).

It is common for a single-base substitution to alter the coding sequence. If the base-pair change results in a codon that codes for a different amino acid, this is known as a missense mutation. An example of this is if the first base of a codon encoding lysine were to be changed from an A to a G (i.e. AAA/AAG to GAA/GAG); then the amino acid encoded would change to a glutamine. If the amino acid substituted in the protein is chemically very similar − with a similar charge or side chain − the change to the protein may not be that significant (Lewin, 2004). If a radically different amino acid is substituted, especially in an important region of the protein molecule, the change can be quite serious. The type of single-base substitution that makes the most significant change to a protein's structure is known as a nonsense mutation. Such a mutation produces an early stop codon, prematurely terminating the translation and leading to a potentially shortened protein. An example of this would be if the last base of a tyrosine codon were mutated from a C or a U to a G or an A (i.e. UAC/UAU to UAA/UAG), producing a stop codon in this part of the message. How much of the protein was actually produced would depend on how near to the start of the transcript this mutation occurred (Strachan and Read, 1999).

INSERTIONS AND DELETIONS

Nucleotides inserted into or deleted from coding regions of DNA can have very serious consequences for a gene, whether a single base is lost or gained, or larger sections of DNA are transposed from another locus. As each specific codon consists of a triplet of nucleotides, the addition of a single nucleotide will lead to a frameshift effect, with each subsequent codon being read wrongly. This shift in the translational reading frame will often lead to the introduction of a premature termination codon, causing a similar effect to a nonsense mutation. Larger insertions or deletions will add or remove large portions of coding sequence, as well as potentially causing a frameshift, unless the number of nucleotides gained or lost is a multiple of three, in which case the reading frame is not altered (Lewin, 2004) (Figure 7.1).

Normal sequence

mRNA   AGA CCA AAG UAC AUU AGG...

protein   Arg - Pro - Lys - Tyr - Ile - Arg ...

Missense mutation

A to G substitution

↓

mRNA   AGA CCA **G**AG UAC AUU AGG ...

protein   Arg - Pro - Glu - Tyr - Ile - Arg - ...

Nonsense mutation

A to G substitution

↓

mRNA   AGA CCA AAG UA**G** AUU AGG ...

protein   Arg - Pro - Lys - STOP

Termination

1bp Insertion

Insertion of C

↓   Frameshift

mRNA   AGA CCA A**C**A GUA CAU UAG G ...

protein   Arg - Pro - Thr - Val - His - STOP

Termination

Figure 7.1   Some types of mutation.

GENETIC DISEASE

Germline (germ cells) mutations accumulate over the generations and have either a neutral or a harmful (pathogenic) effect on an organism. Mutations that are disadvantageous to an organism are slowly removed from the general population by natural selection, but this can take many, many generations. These harmful mutations can give rise to various genetic diseases (Strachan and Read, 1999). Over the past decade or so, more and more diseases have been linked to genetic alterations. Monogenic disorders, caused by a mutation in a single gene, have been the simplest to understand and identify. Genes such as the one for dystrophin, linked to Duchenne muscular dystrophy, or *CFTR,* linked to cystic fibrosis, have been found to be altered in patients with these diseases (Strachan and Read, 1999). Mutations in these essential genes alter their functions, and patients with mutations in both chromosomal copies of these genes are unable to produce fully functional protein. These are recessive genetic disorders, and those people with only a single mutant allele are not affected. Some genetic disorders are dominant, with a mutant form of the protein having such a harmful (often toxic) effect on a patient that only a single mutant copy of the gene is needed to produce it. An example of this is the *HD* gene, which plays a role in Huntington's disease (Gusella and MacDonald, 1993).

Much more complicated are polygenic disorders, diseases that are significantly affected by combinations of many disease susceptibility genes (along with environmental contributions) acting together. Diseases such as diabetes and some forms of heart disease are thought to act in a manner similar to this. Harmful genes have a cumulative effect, and if several genes associated with a particular disease act together they will increase the susceptibility of an individual to that disease (Strachan and Read, 1999).

CANCER AS A GENETIC DISEASE

It is known that cancer is linked to harmful genetic alterations of cells, and many genes have been linked to various forms of cancer, but the genetics of cancer is very complicated and less well understood than classic genetics. No single cancer-causing gene that is mutated in all cancers has ever been discovered, and even in specific types of cancer there can be several possible genetic mechanisms and genes involved in the formation of a tumour. In some families, an inherited disposition has been shown to play a role in cancer formation, but these familial cancers make up only a small proportion of cancer cases (Ponder, 2001).

Cancer is a collection of disorders sharing the common feature of uncontrolled cell growth, which leads to the formation of a mass of cells known as a 'neoplasm' or 'tumour'. Malignant neoplasms have the ability to invade adjacent tissues and often metastasize to more distant parts of the body, a process that is the cause of

90% of cancer deaths (Sporn, 1996). There are more than 200 types of cancer, and each is classified according to the tissue type in which it arises.

Cancers are almost always derived from a single ancestral somatic cell. The cells in an emerging neoplasm accumulate a series of genetic changes that lead to changes in gene activity and phenotype (Ponder, 2001). From studies on the incidence of cancer, it is thought that up to six or seven events are needed to turn a normal cell into a fully-fledged invasive carcinoma. This is initially very confusing, because the probability of a single cell undergoing six independent mutations is virtually nil. But there are mechanisms that explain how this process can happen. Altered cells are subject to selection, and eventually a cell population evolves that can escape the controls of proliferation and territory. The first mutations increase proliferation (growth), and this gives an increased target population of cells for the next mutation. At the same time, some mutations will alter the stability of the whole genome, at either the DNA or chromosome level, and increase the overall mutation rate. This is a multistep process, which explains why tumours always develop in stages, from benign growths to malignant tumour cells, at each step developing new mutations (Kinzler and Vogelstein, 1996).

Cancer-causing mutations generally affect genes that regulate cellular growth (the cell cycle − see Chapter 4) or cell death (apoptosis). It is thought that this process involves up to six essential alterations in cell physiology, including: self-sufficiency in the production of positive growth signals; disregard of inhibitory growth signals; an acquired capability for sustained growth (immortality of the cell); angiogenesis (blood vessel development); and finally metastasis (invasion and spread). Each of these changes represents the breaching of one of the body's anticancer mechanisms. These are predominantly somatic events, although in many of the inherited cancer syndromes one of these events may be inherited. Mutagenic environmental factors such as diet, radiation and exposure to carcinogenic compounds (e.g. cigarette smoke) can also affect the probability of these mutational events (Jorde et al., 2000).

The regulatory components that give the signals for cellular growth or inhibition of growth are usually external growth factors, acting via complex signalling pathways. It is various members of these pathways, as well as cell-cycle components, that are inactivated or down- or up-regulated in many of the tumorigenic alterations to cell physiology. Growth signals include cellular growth factors such as platelet-derived growth factor (PDGF) and transforming growth factor α (TGFα). Their signalling pathways are altered by many cancers to allow self-sufficiency in growth (Hanahan and Weinberg, 2000). Antigrowth signals include growth factors such as TGFβ, and these need to be inactivated to allow cancer progression. These growth inhibitory signals are received by receptor molecules on the cell surface and coupled to other complicated networks of signalling pathways. Many of these signals are associated with the cell cycle, and can force cells out of the active proliferative cycle into a dormant state, where they remain until signalled at some future point. There are other complicated pathways governing apoptosis, senescence and angiogenesis, which all have to be overcome in the development of a cancer (Hanahan and Weinberg, 2000). Once the cell has become hyperproliferative and cancerous, metastasis is a further multistep process, in which the tumour cells have to detach from the primary tumour site and then reattach (via specific adhesion molecules) to the vascular tissues or other tissue sites to be invaded. Extracellular matrix proteins have to be degraded by enzymes released from the tumour or the surrounding cells (Chambers and Matrisian, 1997).

The multistage theory of cancer has become further complicated with the recent discovery of cancer stem cells (Reya *et al.,* 2001). Normal stem cells repair and renew our tissues, but recent research has focused on the idea that these have a kind of 'evil twin', a cancer stem cell (Abbott, 2006). These would make up just a tiny subset of the cells in a cancer, but are proposed to be able to proliferate and self-renew extensively, thus sustaining tumour growth. These cells were first isolated in leukaemias (Bonnet and Dick, 1997), but have now also been found in some solid tumours, including brain (Clarke, 2004) and prostate (Collins *et al.,* 2005) cancers. This has very important implications for treatment as, rather as a weed can grow back from its roots, it is very conceivable that only the eradication of these cells can lead to an effective cancer cure. Cancer stem cells might arise from the mutational transformation of normal stem cells, while in other cases mutations might cause non-stem cells cells to acquire stem cell properties (Pardal, Clarke and Morrison, 2003).

Cancer genes can be divided into three main groups, according to whether they activate cellular proliferation (oncogenes), inhibit proliferation (tumour suppressors) or participate in DNA repair (Strachan and Read, 1999).

ONCOGENES

Oncogenes were the first cancer-causing genes to be identified; they activate cellular proliferation, leading to unregulated cell growth and differentiation (Ponder, 2001). Most oncogenes are derived from a non-mutant version of the gene known as a 'proto-oncogene', which is usually involved in normal cellular growth. When a mutation occurs in a proto-oncogene, it can become transformed to form an oncogene (Varmus, 1985). Oncogenes can also be introduced from several types of DNA and RNA (retrovirus) virus, which can integrate mutant oncogenes into the genome of a host. Oncogenes are usually dominant and activated by 'gain-of-function mutations'. Germline mutations in oncogenes are very uncommon, so this is predominantly a somatic event. Examples of oncogenes include *ras, myc, abl, fos* and *jun.* The gene *ras* is known to be mutated in up to 15% of all cancers (Davies *et al.,* 2002).

TUMOUR SUPPRESSOR GENES

Tumour suppressor genes are 'anti-oncogenes', inhibiting cellular proliferation; they are usually inactivated by 'loss-of-function mutations' in cancer development (Ponder, 2001). The first evidence for these loss-of-function genetic changes came from studies in the rare childhood eye cancer retinoblastoma. From studying sporadic and familial retinoblastoma, in 1971 Knudson formulated his two-hit model of carcinogenesis. In the familial form of the cancer, an affected parent has a 50% chance of passing the condition to an offspring, and this is usually bilateral (in both eyes), whereas the sporadic form has no additional risk of inheritance and is usually in one eye only. Knudson hypothesized that this must be a two-hit event, with two rate-limiting steps for tumour formation.

In the inherited form, this is now known to result in predisposition to tumour formation because of germline mutations in one of the two copies of the tumour suppressor gene (Macleod, 2000). Somatic mutation of the second copy of the gene during the individual's lifetime results in tumour progression and formation. The second hit can be by point mutation, by larger areas of chromosomal loss (allelic loss), or by other methods of silencing the gene. In the sporadic form, two separate sporadic 'hits' are needed in the same cell for it to develop into a tumour clone. The minuscule chance of this rare event happening in both eyes is why formation of sporadic bilateral cancer is an incredibly unlikely event (Knudson, 1971) (Figure 7.2).

The gene involved, *RB1*, which encodes the cell-cycle regulatory protein pRb, has now been discovered on chromosome 13q14. Other important tumour suppressor genes include *p53*, *p16*, *BRCA*-1, *BRCA*-2 and *PTEN* (Jorde *et al.*, 2000). The *p53* gene *TP53* is known to be the most mutated gene involved in human cancer, with key roles in cell cycle control, apoptosis, angiogenesis and genetic stability. As it has such a central role in so many cancer-controlling pathways and activities, this is probably the single most important tumour suppressor gene, and does not function correctly in most human cancers. In around half of these tumours, *p53* is inactivated by mutations in *TP53* (Vogelstein, Lane and Levine, 2000).

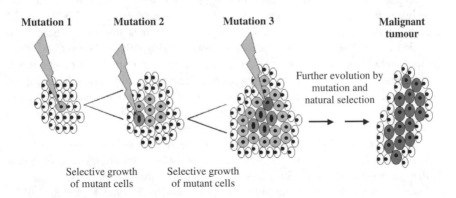

Figure 7.2 The multistage evolution of a cancer, with successive mutations giving cells a growth advantage; expanded populations of cells thus present a larger target for the next mutation. Cells are shaded progressively darker after each mutation.

DNA REPAIR GENES

The final class of gene implicated in carcinogenesis is involved in the various DNA repair mechanisms that allow accurate DNA replication. In some inherited disorders and familial cancer syndromes, defects in these repair mechanisms lead to genomic instability. Genomic instability leads to chromosomal abnormalities such as breaks, abnormal chromosome numbers and widespread mutations; these somatic changes often affect genes that are important in proliferation and carcinogenesis (Jorde *et al.,* 2000). Several colorectal and gastric cancer syndromes are known to have defects in the replication of short tandem repeat sequences (microsatellite sequences), known as microsatellite instability. This replication error defect is caused by mutations in the mismatch repair genes *MLH1* and *MSH2*, which lead to a cascade of secondary mutations in oncogenes and tumour suppressor genes, giving rise to cancer (Loeb, 1994). These replication error defects are also seen in some cases of sporadic cancer.

Chromosomal instability is seen in a larger number of cancers where there are abnormal numbers of chromosomes or smaller regions of chromosomal loss/gain or rearrangement. This process may be related to a mitotic checkpoint involving the *hBUB1* gene (Cahill *et al.,* 1998), and can be stimulated by processes that affect the three-dimensional structure of the DNA molecule, such as ultraviolet radiation and chemical mutagens (Breivik and Gaudernack, 1999), and promote abnormal DNA repair. Chromosomal abnormalities increase during the progression of a cancer and lead to further alterations in cell physiology.

METHYLATION IN TUMOURIGENESIS

Evidence has been accumulating which suggests that the methylation of cytosine bases has an important role in gene silencing (Antequera, Boyes and Bird, 1990). This 'epigenetic' mechanism of gene inactivation has now been discovered to play an increasingly great role in carcinogenesis (Baylin and Herman, 2000). In the mammalian genome, methylation occurs only at cytosines that are located 5′ to guanosine bases, known as the CpG dinucleotide (Bird, 1992). These CpG dinucleotides have been successively depleted in the human genome over its evolution, a phenomenon referred to as CG suppression. The remaining CpGs have a high frequency of methylation. This is thought to facilitate the repression of 'parasitic' repeated regions of the genome, such as retroviral genomic elements and self-replicating DNA junk regions, known as transposons.

In contrast to the CG suppression seen in the mammalian genome, there are small regions of DNA 300–3000 bp in length where the frequency of CpGs is either at expected values or higher. These areas are known as CpG islands and they are protected from methylation (Gardiner-Garden and Frommer, 1987). CpG islands represent roughly 1–2% of the genome, and are located close to the promoter regions of roughly half of all human genes (Antequera, Boyes and Bird, 1990). The methylation of promoters and internal CpG sites silences the gene with which it is associated. This occurs in the promoters of selected genes and on the inactivated X-chromosome of females. It also plays a role in genomic imprinting, whereby genes are expressed differently on maternal and paternal chromosomes as a result of differences in DNA methylation between the parental alleles (Reik and Walter, 2001). This silencing is permanent and transmitted through mitosis (Baylin, Belinsky and Herman, 2000).

With some exceptions, CpG islands located in the promoter or the inside of active genes should be unmethylated. This is why aberrant methylation in the promoters of normally active genes has an important role in loss-of-gene function. The first two genes shown to have aberrant CpG island promoter methylation in cancer were the gene for calcitonin (CALCA) and *MyoD*. Since then, CpG island methylation has been observed in other tumour suppressor genes known to be involved in cancers, including E-cadherin, *hMLH1*, *BRCA*-1, *pRb*, *p16Ink4a* and *p14ARF* (Baylin and Herman, 2000).

The consequences of methylation are known, but the exact mechanism responsible in aberrant methylation is poorly understood. The main DNA methyltransferase enzyme DNMT1 works during DNA replication by recognizing methylated CpG sites on the parent strand and methylates correlating cytosines on the daughter strand. This enzyme, or other enzymes that work in a similar manner, may be functioning incorrectly in certain cancer cells (Rhee *et al.*, 2000) (Figure 7.3).

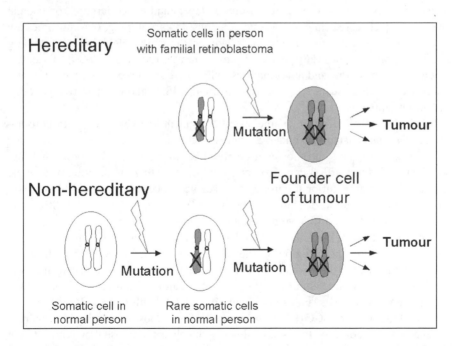

Figure 7.3 Knudson's two-hit hypothesis: tumour formation in both hereditary and non-hereditary retinoblastoma. A one-hit clone is a precursor to the tumour in non-hereditary retinoblastomas, whereas all cells are one-hit clones in hereditary retinoblastoma.

Unlike genetic mutation, inactivation of a gene by promoter methylation is potentially reversible by demethylating drugs. Compounds based on the demethylating agent 5-aza-2'-deoxycytidine (Decitabine) may form the basis of a new class of anticancer drugs in methylation-positive tumours.

IDENTIFYING CANCER GENES

There are many ways to identify the genetic abnormalities that develop during the progression of a cancer. Chromosomal loss and rearrangements and deletions of smaller regions of the chromosome give clues to the locations of many of the abnormal genes involved in carcinogenesis. Candidate tumour suppressor genes in these regions can be screened for inactivating mutations or methylation (Strachan and Read, 1999).

DEFINING CHROMOSOMAL ABNORMALITIES IN A TUMOUR

Karyotyping is used to count chromosome numbers and to see large chromosomal alterations, such as rearrangements and deletions. In karyotyping, chromosomes are analysed by culturing the tumour cells, adding the drug colchicine and staining and photographing the now visible chromosomes (Jorde *et al.*, 2000). To detect much smaller deletions and abnormalities, other more sensitive techniques are used. These include fluorescence *in situ* hybridization (FISH) and comparative genomic hybridization (CGH).

In FISH, a labelled chromosome-specific segment is hybridized with chromosomal DNA and visualized under a fluorescence microscope. This technique can tell whether there is a chromosomal deletion, because the labelled probe will not be able to hybridize. FISH can also determine whether there is deletion of a single chromosome or an additional chromosome segment, because it is possible to visualize how many locations the probe hybridizes (Trask, 1991). The use of differently coloured probes has led to several variations of this technique.

With CGH, tumour DNA and normal DNA are labelled with different colours and then hybridized together. Regions of the tumour DNA with deletions or duplications that are not present in the normal DNA will give a different colour balance, allowing the detection of multiple abnormal chromosomal regions (Kallioniemi *et al.*, 1992). This technology has been updated by combining CGH with microarray technology (see later) to form array-CGH. This gives the ability to look at genetic abnormalities in cancers at a genome-wide level, while being much easier to use than conventional CGH, and also increases the sensitivity and resolution (Kashiwagi and Uchida, 2000).

Another method of screening for small areas of chromosomal imbalance is allelic imbalance analysis. In this technique, highly variable repeat markers in the chromosomal region of interest, known as microsatellites, are screened in both tumour and normal tissue. If one of the heterozygous markers (multiple repeats) in the normal tissue becomes homozygous (a single repeat) in the tumour, this suggests that an allele has been lost, and there is a deletion in this region. This is known as loss of heterozygosity (LOH) or allelic loss. Alleles can also be gained, through chromosomal duplications (Strachan and Read, 1999).

MUTATIONAL ANALYSIS

To detect relatively large deletions in a gene, Southern blotting is usually used. In this technique, a labelled DNA probe is hybridized to a DNA fragment of interest that has been transferred to a nylon membrane (Southern, 1975). This technique has evolved with the production of DNA chips, or microarrays, whereby thousands of tiny DNA fragments are attached to a solid substrate (usually glass or silicon) and then probed with a known gene or fragment. This allows the monitoring of expression levels or mutations in thousands of genes simultaneously (Khan *et al.,* 1999). This technology is still comparatively expensive, but has now got to the stage where it is possible to screen every gene in the genome in a very rapid period of time. Gene-chips that are able to simultaneously screen hundreds of thousands of well-characterized mutations are now available, but these are very expensive, do not detect novel mutations not present on the chip and are not yet cost effective for routine use (Wadman, 2006). For deletions under 50 bp in size, and other small genetic alterations, the most sensitive way of screening genes of interest is still direct DNA sequencing. DNA sequencer machine technology, developed for the various genome sequencing projects, has greatly improved in terms of speed and cost, but when one needs to screen multiple genes in many tumour samples it can still be too technically demanding, costly and time-consuming. This is why pre-screening techniques are often used to pick out a sample that definitely contains a mutation. The region of interest is amplified by using a technique known as polymerase chain reaction (PCR) (Strachan and Read, 1999).

POLYMERASE CHAIN REACTION

Polymerase chain reaction is a rapid and versatile method for amplifying a defined target DNA sequence within a source of DNA. Some prior knowledge of the DNA sequence of the target is needed and, from this sequence information, two oligonucleotide primers are designed that will hybridize to this sequence and surround the area to be amplified. When the DNA template is denatured (heated to form single-stranded DNA), these primers anneal and bind to the specific complementary DNA sequences at the target site. In the presence of a heat-resistant DNA polymerase enzyme and DNA precursor nucleotides, these primers can initiate the synthesis of new DNA strands, which are complementary to the DNA strands of the target DNA. PCR is called a chain reaction because the newly synthesized DNA acts as a template for further DNA synthesis in subsequent cycles. After about 25 cycles of DNA synthesis, the products of the PCR will include about 10^5 copies of the specific target sequence. The PCR products can then be visualized using agarose gel electrophoresis. This technique uses the fact that, since DNA is a charged molecule, it can migrate through a porous gel when a current is passed through it. This allows DNA fragments to be separated according to size (Sambrook and Russell, 2001).

Used as an alternative to Southern blotting, reverse-transcriptase PCR (RT-PCR) is a technique for amplifying RNA molecules. The RNA strand is first 'reverse transcribed', using a reverse-transcriptase (RT) enzyme, into its complementary DNA sequence. The resulting DNA is then amplified by PCR. Quantitative PCR (qPCR) is a modification of the PCR technique used to rapidly measure the quantity of the PCR product (Bustin, 2005). This is preferably done in real time (confusingly also known as RT-PCR), and is an indirect method for quantitatively measuring starting amounts of DNA or RNA. Real-time PCR has been developed from the application of fluorescence techniques to RT-PCR, using instrumentation that combines amplification, detection and quantification. The PCR product fluoresces, and the amount of product present can be measured by the amount of light produced. Real-time PCR is often used to determine whether a genetic sequence is present and, if it is present, to determine the number of copies in the sample (Bustin, 2005).

PRE-SCREENING TECHNIQUES

After amplifying an area of interest in the gene using PCR, the PCR products screened for genetic alterations by using techniques such as SSCP conformational polymorphism), DGGE (denaturing gradient gel electrophoresis) and DHPLC (denaturing high-performance liquid chromatography) analysis. SSCP and DGGE are both gel-based techniques which make use of the fact that certain conditions alter the rate of migration of DNA fragments in gel electrophoresis. DHPLC uses a similar technique, but DNA fragments are instead separated on an HPLC column and detected using computer software (Xiao and Oefner, 2001).

GENETIC SCREENING OF CANCER

As cancer has a strong genetic basis, genetic screening should potentially have applications for determining prognostic information. In classic monogenic (one gene) familial genetic disorders such as Huntington's disease, screening of potentially affected family members can allow them to know what their chances are of developing a disease (Strachan and Read, 1999). Screening can also allow potential parents to know what the likelihood is of any future offspring developing the condition. Unfortunately, in cancer studies screening is not so straightforward, as a result of the complexity of cancer genetics. Inherited cancer syndromes that act similarly to classic genetic diseases cause only about 1% of human cancer (Ponder, 2001). A further 5−10% of all cancers (depending on how strictly defined) have a more general familial basis (Ponder, 2001). In these families, several cases of common cancers are found, usually falling into general groups of cancers (e.g. breast and ovary, or colon, endometrium and urinary). Only these rarer familial cancers have a requirement for genetic screening. If the risk to a family member can be determined, there is a possibility that preventive steps can be taken.

So far, the most common cancer syndrome screened for is familial breast and ovarian cancer caused by the genes *BRCA*-1 and *BRCA*-2, and many clinical cancer centres as well as private companies now offer screening for *BRCA*-1 and *BRCA*-2 mutations in families with multiple cases of these tumours (Foster *et al.*, 2002). If mutations are found, it is estimated that a woman has up to an 85% lifetime risk of developing breast cancer and a 60% risk of developing ovarian cancer (Armstrong, Eisen and Weber, 2000). If *BRCA* mutations are detected, intensive monitoring can be used to pick up developing tumours at an early stage. For the most high-risk cases, preventive measures such as prophylatic mastectomy or administering drugs that reduce the chances of developing these cancers (such as tamoxifen), can be considered. Unfortunately, *BRCA*-1 and *BRCA*-2 mutation-associated familial cases account for only around 15−20% of familial cancers, so it is possible there are many genetic risk factors yet to be discovered (Balmain, 2001).

Genes that confer strong susceptibility to other familial cancers are also starting to be screened for in a similar manner. Genetic testing can now be used to confirm diagnosis or to predict disease development in families potentially affected by the many of the better-studied but relatively rare cancer syndromes (e.g. retinoblastoma, Li-Fraumeni syndrome and Von Hippel-Lindau syndrome) which are caused by single gene defects and have clear patterns of inheritance (Hampel *et al.*, 2004). Screening programmes are being developed and starting to be offered commercially and by some hospitals for other useful genes strongly involved in more general familial cancer syndromes. These include the *p16Ink4a* gene in familial skin melanoma, and the various tumour-suppressor and DNA-repair genes involved in the familial colon cancer syndromes, such as familial adenomatous polyposis (FAP) and hereditary non-polyposis colon cancer (HNPCC). These genes significantly increase the risk of getting the cancer and detection of these mutations indicates that better surveillance and/or the deployment of early prophylactic measures may be appropriate (Rogowski, 2006).

FUTURE APPLICATIONS OF CANCER GENETICS: CHEMOSENSITIVITY AND GENE THERAPY

Aside from the application of genetic screening in the small number of familial cancers, genetic technologies will have increasingly more applications in the research and treatment of cancer in the future. By defining the genetic abnormalities and alterations in specific types of cancer, we have massively increased our understanding of how these tumours develop, helping us to understand how to target and fight them, and at the same time to discover new drug targets. The closer that specific tumour cells have been studied, the more genetic abnormalities and differences in their genetic profiles have been discovered, even in cells that are supposedly from the same tumour type. Techniques such as DNA microchips or microarrays are allowing us to profile simultaneously many of the genetic changes from tumour to tumour. The more we understand how certain tumours with certain molecular profiles behave, the more we will be able specifically to tailor treatments for them. Eventually we will be able to develop bespoke drug regimens for specific tumours, minimizing drug resistance and side effects.

GENE THERAPY

Ultimately the best way of treating a cancer would be to find a way of genetically modifying the tumour cells, correcting the genetic defect. This technique is known as 'gene therapy', and currently much research is going into developing potential mechanisms for delivering genes to target cells, inhibiting the expression of specific genes and correcting genetic defects. This technology is a still a long way from becoming a useful clinical treatment, but has such great potential for the future that it has to be discussed here. There have been several potential gene delivery systems discovered to date, and possible vectors currently being studied include attenuated DNA and RNA viruses that integrate part of their genome (containing the target gene) into a target cell. These viruses have had most of their viral genes removed to stop them replicating, but there are still safety and immunological problems with the technique. Non-viral vectors that avoid these problems are also currently in development, including liposome vector systems, but these have a lower efficiency of gene transfer and do not integrate genes into the chromosome, so gene expression is for a shorter duration (Strachan and Read, 1999).

Recessive monogenic disorders are the diseases most amenable to being treated with this technique, because only small amounts of introduced gene product can potentially have an effect. Trials have been carried out on diseases including adenosine deaminase deficiency (ADA), cystic fibrosis and familial hypercholesterolaemia. The use of gene therapy technologies to treat cancers is potentially more complicated, because a cancer cell can have several different genes mutated. Tumour cells are constantly being selected against, and evolve resistance to, various treatments, so such problems would need to be overcome if this technique were to be used as a cancer therapy.

Different strategies have been tested in many cancer types, including pancreatic (Halloran *et al.,* 2000), colorectal (Kerr, 2003) and breast cancers (Takahashi *et al.,* 2006). Strategies have included the addition of copies of working tumour suppressor genes or the suppression of oncogenes, protection of bone marrow against chemotherapy by the addition of drug resistance genes, enhancement of the immunological response against a tumour and attempts to enable targeted cell death. A first potential breakthrough for this experimental form of treatment involved removing immune cells from melanoma sufferers and genetically engineering them to better recognize the cancer when reintroduced into the patients (Morgan *et al.,* 2006). Further studies targeting cell death have involved the genetic introduction into the tumour of an enzyme that can convert non-toxic drug precursors into toxic forms that will selectively kill the tumour cells without any side effects. These are a very promising start, but much more research is needed to improve the targeting of this technology, and to increase the efficiency, gene uptake and safety. Despite these problems, gene therapy has enormous potential for the future of medicine.

CONCLUSION

Cancer, like most diseases, is caused to a greater or lesser extent by a combination of the actions of genes and the environment (Strachan and Read, 1999). In the last few decades, the human genome project and the enormous improvements in molecular biology and genomic technologies have enormously increased our understanding of

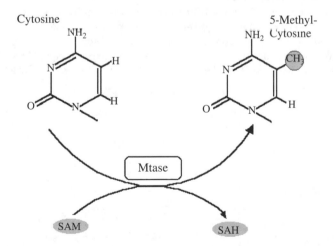

Figure 7.4 The DNA methyltransferase enzyme catalysing the addition of a methyl (CH_3) group on to a cytosine base, and using *S*-adenosyl methionine (SAM) as a methyl donor. SAH: *S*-adenosyl homocysteine.

the genetic abnormalities and defects underlying cancer progression (Balmain *et al.*, 2003). This is already having enormous benefits in the screening and treatment of many types of cancer. Utilizing this knowledge to provide treatments and therapies for the great majority of common (sporadic) cancers is likely going to take a very long time (Ponder, 2001).

To give an example, since the early 1980s evidence has accumulated that the oncogene EGFR is overexpressed in many tumours, with up to a third of epithelial tumours expressing high levels, and with high expression correlating with poor prognosis (Ozanne *et al.*, 1986). The EGFR gene was first characterized and cloned in 1984 (Downward *et al.*, 1984), but it has subsequently taken nearly 20 years for treatments to be developed and licensed that target this gene (Arteaga, 2001) and its family members, such as HER2 (Menard *et al.*, 2003). This new generation of anticancer drugs includes the EGFR inhibitor molecules Gefitinib and Erlotinib (Blackledge and Averbuch, 2004) and the anti-HER2 monoclonal antibody Herceptin (Bell, 2002; and see also Chapter 10). This demonstrates that while there is enormous potential for new cancer treatments and therapies developed from this explosion in our understanding of the genetics of cancer, patience is needed for these new therapies to reach the clinic (Figure 7.4).

FURTHER SOURCES

Bartlett, J.M. (2002) Approaches to the analysis of gene expression using mRNA: a technical overview. *Mol Biotechnol*, **21**, 149—60.

Chung, C.H., Bernard, P.S. and Perou, C.M. (2002) Molecular portraits and the family tree of cancer. *Nat Genet*, **32**(Suppl), 533—40.

Goldberg, J.I. and Borgen, P.I. (2006) Breast cancer susceptibility testing: past, present and future. *Expert Review of Anticancer Therapy*, **8**, 1205—14.

Lewin, B. (2004) *GenesVIII*, Oxford University Press, Oxford.

Stewart, B.W. and PaulKleihues, P. (eds) (2003) *World Cancer Report*, IARC Press.

Strachan, T. and Read, A.P. (1999) *Human Molecular Genetics II*, BIOS Scientific Publishers, Oxford.

8 The Immune System

HELMOUT MODJTAHEDI AND AILSA CLARKE

BACKGROUND

The human body is constantly assaulted by a variety of pathogens such as bacteria, viruses, fungi and parasites. These pathogens vary in shape and size (from $20\,\mu m$ (viruses) up to 7 m (tapeworms)) and cause diseases and cancers in different ways. Our body has evolved three kinds of defence strategy against these foreign invaders and other antigens: (i) physical (e.g. intact skin and mucosa) and chemical (e.g. acid in stomach) barriers; (ii) natural (also called innate or non-specific) immune responses (e.g. phagocytosis); and (iii) adaptive (also called acquired or specific) immune responses. In the majority of cases, the destruction of invading pathogens is successfully achieved by the first two lines of body defence. If it is not, however, the third line of defence, the adaptive response, will activate against the invaders (Figure 8.1). Adaptive immune responses against pathogens are mediated by a special group of immune cells called lymphocytes. The activation, proliferation and differentiation of different types of lymphocyte, through either the antibody-mediated immune response (AMI) or cell-mediated immune response (CMI), results in the elimination of the invading pathogens. Once the infection is cleared, most of the expanded population of antigen-specific lymphocytes undergoes programmed cell death, while a small number of these lymphocytes differentiate into long-lived memory lymphocytes, which remain in the circulation for decades after the first exposure to a particular pathogen. As a result, when the body encounters the same pathogen a second time, it is destroyed very rapidly (within hours) and efficiently by the memory cells. In such situations, the individual is said to have developed immunity or specific resistance against that pathogen. But the pathogens have also developed various strategies (e.g. mutation or down-regulation of immunogenic antigens) to overcome the body defences (Abbass and Lichtman, 2006), so there is a constant battle between the invader and the host.

In addition to its primary role in fighting infectious agents, it is clear that the immune system plays an important role in a number of pathological conditions. For example, abnormal immune responses against a harmless substance (e.g. food, pollen) or self-antigens have been associated with allergies and autoimmune diseases. Normal immune responses against a tissue or organ transplant from an

The Biology of Cancer, Second Edition. Edited by J. Gabriel
© 2007 John Wiley & Sons, Ltd.

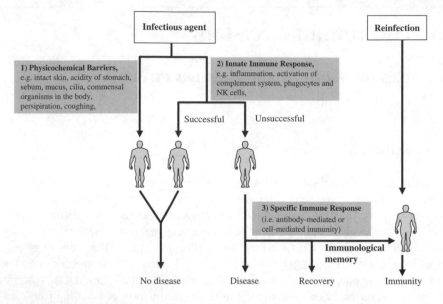

Figure 8.1 Three different strategies used by the body against foreign pathogens. The first two lines of defences are usually sufficient to eliminate infectious agents. If not, the body recovers as a result of activation of the adaptive immune responses, which generate specific populations of lymphocytes against the invading pathogens. Some of these lymphocytes remain in circulation as memory cells and provide immunity against reinfection by the original antigen. The principle of vaccination is to alter the antigen in a way that prevents it causing disease but stimulates production of memory B-lymphocytes or memory T-lymphocytes against such antigens.

incompatible individual are associated with transplant rejection (Buckley, 2003). The immune cells in transplanted organs and tissues may also attack and destroy the tissues of the host, causing graft-versus-host disease (Gulbahce *et al.*, 2003).

There are convincing lines of evidence that suggest a fully functional immune system can prevent the incidence of cancer. Cancer incidence, along with incidence of infectious diseases, increases rapidly in old age (see Chapter 1) as the ability of the immune system to recognize and provoke a strong immune response against pathogens declines (Franceschi, Bonafe and Valensin, 2000; Effros, 2003). The incidence of cancer has also been shown to increase in immunosuppressed patients, such as patients treated with cytotoxic drugs and AIDS (acquired immune deficiency syndrome) patients (Appay and Rowland-Jones, 2002; Vial and Descotes, 2003).

In general, as cancer cells are almost identical to healthy body cells, the immune system is less efficient at dealing with tumours than with infectious agents. Indeed, the majority of human antigens are tumour-associated antigens and are expressed in lower amounts in normal cells. In recent years, as a result of our better understanding of the cells and molecules of the immune system, the identification and characterization of tumour antigens of biological and clinical significance and the development of novel adjuvants, we have been able to manipulate the immune system and provoke immune responses against human tumour antigens that are not normally immunogenic in cancer patients. Several clinical trials are currently underway in cancer patients using tumour cells transfected with genes for cytokines and other co-stimulatory molecules, tumour antigens or antigen fragments in combination with new adjuvants, to find a source of cancer vaccines (Moingeon, 2001; Romero *et al.*, 2002). Monoclonal antibodies have been developed against human tumour antigens and some of these antibodies are currently used for the management of human cancers (see Chapter 10).

In this chapter, an account of the cells and molecules of the normal immune system will be presented, giving details of their functions. The relationship between the immune system and cancer, novel immunotherapeutic strategies (e.g. cancer vaccines) for human cancers and the effects of cytotoxic drugs on the immune system will then be discussed.

THE FIRST LINE OF BODY DEFENCE

Our body has evolved three kinds of defence strategy against infectious agents, some of which (i.e. viruses) have been associated with the development of human cancers (Marieb and Hoehn, 2007). All viruses, and some bacteria, can live and multiply inside the host cells. These are called intracellular pathogens. In contrast, most bacteria and larger parasites live and multiply outside the cells, in the body tissues and fluids. These are called extracelluar pathogens. The first line of defence against infectious agents is non-immunological and involves a number of physical and chemical barriers, also called external defences. An unbroken skin is the most important protection for the body, acting as a physical barrier to stop invasion by foreign micro-organisms and other substances. The skin also has secretions, such as acidic sweat and fatty acids from oil glands, which can destroy or inhibit bacterial growth on its surface. In addition, there is a normal population of microflora which can colonize the surface of the skin and inhibit growth of potential pathogens by competing for the available space and nutrients at the site (Wood, 2006).

Mucous membranes at the openings to the digestive, respiratory, urinary and reproductive tracts also protect the body from invasion by foreign micro-organisms. Mucous traps bacteria and other foreign substances and can be expelled from the body. The urinary and reproductive tracts are free from micro-organisms under normal circumstances. Regular urination and secretion of mucous flushes any micro-organisms towards the outside of the body, although some microflora and opportunistic pathogens can enter from the surrounding areas. Movement of the gut contents and expulsion of the faeces helps to remove unwanted bacteria.

Other physical and chemical barriers include the anti-microbial enzyme lysozyme in perspiration, tears, saliva and nasal secretions, and the acidity of gastric juice in the stomach (Wood, 2006; Marieb and Hoehn, 2007). Such physical and chemical barriers are often sufficient in preventing the infection and disease caused by pathogens (Figure 8.1).

THE IMMUNE SYSTEM

The immune system is a complex network of immune cells, cytokines, lymphoid tissues and organs that work together to eliminate infectious agents and other antigens (Tables 8.1–8.3). When infectious agents are not stopped by the physical and chemical barriers described above, they enter the body through the skin or mucous membranes. This initiates the first line of immunological defence mechanism, called the innate, non-specific or natural immune response. If the pathogens are not eliminated by the innate immune response then disease ensues and the adaptive, specific or acquired immune response activates, allowing the body to recover (Figure 8.1). The two important differences between the innate and adaptive immune responses are that (i) the latter is highly specific for a particular pathogen/antigen and (ii) the latter response improves with each subsequent exposure to the same antigen. However, as we shall see later on, the innate and adaptive immune responses work together at several levels (e.g. by releasing growth promoting cytokines) in order to destroy invading antigens.

Table 8.1   Cells of the immune system

Cell	Function
Phagocytes	Ingest and digest foreign antigens/pathogens by the process of phagocytosis (e.g. macrophages, neutrophils).
Antigen presenting cells	Process and present antigens to T-lymphocytes (e.g. dendritic cells, macrophages, B-cells).
Natural killer cells	Kill tumour cells and some viral infected cells. Are lymphocytes but, unlike B- and T-cells, lack specificity and memory.
B-lymphocytes	Express antibodies on their cell surface that can bind to antigens and differentiate to antibody-producing plasma cells.
Plasma cells	The antibody secreting form of B-lymphocytes.
Cytotoxic T-cell (killer T-cell, Tc)	Subset of T-lymphocytes (CD8+) that recognize cells expressing foreign antigens in association with MHC-I molecules and kill by releasing cytokines perforin and lymphotoxin. Release other cytokines that stimulate phagocytosis and inhibit viral replication.
Helper T-cell (T_H, T_4)	Subset of T-lymphocytes (CD4+) that produce cytokines to stimulate both antibody and cell-mediated immune response.
Memory T-cells	Develop after the first exposure to a particular antigen. Remain in circulation and recognize the original antigen years after the first exposure, and respond more rapidly and efficiently in second and subsequent exposures.
Suppressor T-cells	Down-regulate the immune responses.

Table 8.2   Important cytokines of the immune system

Cytokine	Function
Interleukin IL-1	Mainly from macrophages, contributing to fever, and T-cell and macrophage activation.
IL-2	Secreted by helper T-cells. Co-stimulate proliferation of helper T-cells, cytotoxic T-cells and B-cells. Activate NK cells.
IL-4	Produced by T- and B-cells and macrophages. Involved in activation of B-cells, differentiation of T_H2-cells and suppression of T_H1-cells
IL-5	Mainly from helper T-cells and mast cells. Principal action in activation and chemoattraction of eosinophils.
IL-6	Mainly from macrophages, endothelial cells and T-cells. Target synthesis of acute phase proteins in the liver. Induce proliferation of antibody producing cells.
IL-8	Macrophage derived chemoattractant for immune system cells and phagocytes to site of inflammation.
IL-10	Secreted by T- and B-cells and macrophages. Involved in suppression of macrophage function and T_H1-cells. Activate B-cells.
IL-12	Produced mainly by dendritic cells and macrophages. Mainly involved in differentiation of T_H1-cells and activation of NK cells and T-cells.
IL-15	Mainly from macrophages. Induce proliferation of NK cells and T-cells.
IL-18	Mainly from macrophages. Enhance NK cytotoxicity and IFN synthesis by T-cells.
Interferons (IFN)	Produced by macrophages, lymphocytes and NK cells. Major macrophage activators. Activate NK cells. Enhance AMI and CMI responses. Antiviral activity.
Tumour necrosis factor (TNF)	Mainly from macrophages and helper T-cells. Cytotoxic to tumour cells. Enhance activity of phagocytic cells.
Lymphotoxin (LT)	Secreted by cytotoxic T-cells. Kills cells by activating cell's own caspase enzymes, which induce an endonuclease to degrade the cell's DNA (apoptosis).
Perforin	Secreted by cytotoxic T-cells and NK cells. Polymerizes to form tubular structures which perforate the lipid bilayer of the target cells, leading to osmotic lysis.
Granzymes	Secreted by cytotoxic T-cells and NK cells. Pass through perforin pores and induce apoptosis from within the target cell cytoplasm.
Transforming growth factor (TGFβ)	Produced by T-cells and monocytes. Inhibits T- and B-cell proliferation and NK cell activity.

INNATE (NATURAL, NON-SPECIFIC) IMMUNE RESPONSE

The innate immune response is present at birth and is mediated by a complex sequence of cellular and molecular events, including phagocytosis, inflammation,

Table 8.3   Important recognition moieties of the immune system

	Function
Antibodies	Produced by plasma cells differentiated from B-lymphocytes. Enhance phagocytosis by opsonization. Neutralize antigens and activate complement. The Ag/Ab complex can bind to effector cells such as NK cells and macrophages, targeting the antigen for destruction by ADCC.
Complement	Over 20 serum glycoproteins that, once activated, lead to cell lysis, inflammation and opsonization.
MHC	Major Histocompatibility Complex molecules bind and 'present' antigenic peptides on the surfaces of cells for recognition by the antigen-specific T-cell receptor (TCR). Two classes: MHC-I on all nucleated cells, MHC-II on antigen presenting immune cells.
CD4	Molecules expressed on helper T-cells bind antigenic peptides presented by MHC-II.
CD8	Molecules expressed on cytotoxic T-cells bind antigenic peptides presented by MHC-I.
Co-stimulatory molecules	Adhesion molecules/cytokines which provide the second signal for T-cell activation.
Antigens/Epitopes	Substances that provoke immune responses (e.g. bacteria, pollen, transplanted tissues) are called antigens. Each antigen may have several components called epitopes, and each epitope provokes the production of a specific antibody or stimulates a specific T-lymphocyte. (Antigen = antibody generator.)
Vaccine	A modified form of the original antigen that is used in vaccination in order to stimulate the production of memory B-cells and memory T-cells without causing the disease. Antigenic preparations that are used in educating the immune system.
Chemotaxis	The migration of a cell to the site of infection in response to a chemical stimulus (e.g. complement components), causing accumulation of leukocytes in inflamed tissues.

complement activation and natural killer cell activation. In contrast to the adaptive immune response, which improves with each successive exposure to the same antigen, the innate immune response does not change following repeated exposures. Some of the main components of the innate immune system, also called innate immunity, are briefly described here.

Phagocytosis and Phagocytic Cells

Phagocytosis is a multistep process by which phagocytic cells engulf and destroy infectious agents. Like other types of white blood cell, phagocytic cells are derived from a common pluripotent stem cell in the red bone marrow. Phagocytes are attracted to the site of infection by a process called chemotaxis. Examples of chemotatic factors include microbial products, damaged leukocytes or tissue cells, complement components (e.g. C5a) and certain cytokines. The process continues with adherence of the phagocyte's plasma membrane to the surface of the micro-organism. This occurs more readily after opsonization, where the microbe is coated by complement proteins or antibody molecules (see below). By extending the plasma membrane projections, called pseudopodia, phagocytic cells engulf the pathogen, forming a phagocytic vacuole (i.e. phagosome), and fuse it with a lysosome. The phagocytosed pathogen can then be digested by the appropriate digestive enzymes (e.g. lysozyme) and bactericidal chemicals. The indigestible products are ejected from the cell by exocytosis. Examples of phagocytic cells include neutrophils, monocytes and macrophages.

Neutrophils, which are the most abundant type of white blood cell, respond very rapidly to infection, are relatively short-lived (1−5 days) and can only phagocytose small pathogens, such as viruses and bacteria. In response to infection, bone marrow can produce between 1 and 2×10^{11} neutrophils per day. The number of neutrophils in the circulation does not alter with age (Lords et al., 2001). In contrast to neutrophils, macrophages ('big eaters') in the tissues are derived from monocytes in the blood, respond more slowly to chemotactic stimuli, but are more efficient in the phagocytosis of the remaining living and dead pathogens. Macrophages can live for months or years and kill infectious agents by several mechanisms; for example, the secretion of a wide range of molecules such as anti-viral interferon or anti-bacterial lysozyme and the generation of oxygen radicals, nitric oxide and chlorine-containing products (Wood, 2006). Macrophages may be fixed in a particular tissue (e.g. kupffer cells in the liver, microglia in the brain) or they may move throughout the body in search of pathogens (these are termed 'wandering macrophages'). The activated macrophages produce a number of cytokines (e.g. Interleukin-1 (IL-1), Interleukin-8 (IL 8), TNFα and IFNα) that stimulate an inflammatory response and bring an additional army of immune cells and molecules to the site of infection (Table 8.2). This additional array of cells and molecules can more effectively destroy the invading pathogens.

Macrophages are also very important in the activation of adaptive (specific) immune responses against invading pathogens, by presenting a fragment of processed antigen on their cell surface in association with class II MHC molecules to CD4+ T-lymphocytes (see later). This results in the activation of CD4+ helper T-lymphocytes, which in turn can stimulate both the antibody-mediated and cell-mediated immune responses against infectious agents (Figure 8.2, and see below).

Inflammation

Damage to the body's tissues by microbial infection, physical agents like heat or sharp objects, and chemical agents such as acid burns, leads to a complex series of non-specific physiological responses, called inflammation. The main aims are to

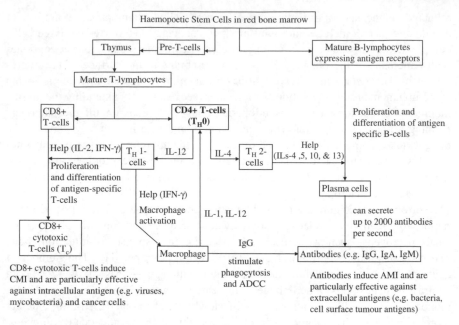

Figure 8.2 The central role played by CD4+ helper T-cells in all types of immune responses. The CD4+ T-cells stimulated by antigen differentiate into CD4+ helper T-cell subsets T_H1 and T_H2. The cytokines released by T_H1-cells in turn help the cell-mediated immune response by increasing the population of antigen specific CD8+ cytotoxic T-cells and by activating macrophages, which are important in the innate immune response. The cytokines released by T_H2-cells can aid the antibody-mediated immune response by increasing the population of antigen specific B-cells and plasma cells. The production of cytokines by macrophages can also activate the proliferation and differentiation of helper T-cells.

localize the infection and prevent the spread of any microbial invaders, to recruit additional immune cells (e.g. neutrophils and monocytes) and molecules from the blood to the infected area, to neutralize toxins and to repair and replace damaged tissue. The tissue macrophages can stimulate inflammation further by releasing cytokines (IL-1, IL-8 and TNFα), which cause vasodilatation, increase vascular permeability and are chemotactic for neutrophils and monocytes (Wood, 2006). Vasodilation increases blood flow to the damaged area, leading to redness and heat at the site of injury. This allows an increase in the concentration of complement and other chemotactic factors at the infected areas, which ultimately enhances phagocyte migration and phagocytosis at the site of injury. Tissue repair can occur once all harmful substances and damage have been removed.

Complement Activation

The complement system contains a cascade of inactive proteins in the blood, which can be activated following the binding of an antibody to bacteria and other foreign cells, or by an alternative pathway involving the presence of bacterial capsular polysaccharides. Once activated, the complement system generates a number of biologically active proteins that enhance inflammation and phagocytosis and promote cell lysis. For example, the complement proteins C3a, C4a and C5a enhance inflammatory reactions by stimulating dilation of arteries, releasing histamine from mast cells and basophils and attracting neutrophils by chemotaxis. Other members of the complement system promote cell lysis by forming the membrane attack complex (C5b–C6, C7, C8 and C9). The complement fragment C3b is an important opsonin and can coat the cell surface of pathogens. Phagocytic cells such as macrophages, monocytes and neutrophils all have C3b receptors on their surface. Such receptors can help the elimination of the pathogens by promoting phagocytosis (Rabson, Roitt and Delves, 2005; Wood, 2006; Marieb and Hoehn, 2007).

Natural Killer (NK) Cells

NK cells are a distinct subpopulation of lymphocytes which play an important role in the natural immune response by mediating cytotoxic effects in the target cells and by releasing cytokines such as IFNγ and TNFα (Tables 8.1 and 8.2). Unlike B- or T-lymphocytes, NK cells lack specificity and memory but can induce spontaneous lysis of cells infected with viruses and of various tumour cells by secretion of perforin and other lytic enzymes (Solana and Mariani, 2000; Rabson, Roitt and Delves, 2005). As described in Chapter 10, NK cells, in addition to their direct cytotoxic killing, can induce an antibody-dependent cell-mediated cytotoxicity (ADCC) in target cells by binding to the Fc portion of the antibody (Gorczynsky and Stanley, 2006). For example, organisms such as protozoa or helminthes, which are too large to be engulfed by phagocytic cells, can be coated with antibodies. When the antigen binding sites of the antibody (e.g human IgG1 and IgG3 antibodies) have bound to such antigens, the Fc portions of the antibodies are free and can bind to the Fc receptor on NK cells, directing cell killing by ADCC (Figure 8.2). In addition to NK cells, macrophages, neutrophils and eosinophils also have Fc receptors that can bind to the Fc portion of the antibody molecule and direct cell killing by ADCC.

While the absolute number of NK cells increases with age, their cytotoxic capacity decreases, and this is a characteristic feature of immunosenescence (Malaguarnera et al., 2001; Rabson, Roitt and Delves, 2005). For example, NK cells from old donors have been shown to respond less efficiently to the mitogenic cytokine IL-2, which can result in decreased proliferation of NK cells and decreased production of IFN by NK cells. This may ultimately lead to a decreased cytotoxic response by NK cells against the target antigen on the infectious agent or tumour cell (Solana and Mariani, 2000).

Cytokines

Both natural and adaptive immunity are coordinated by about 60 cytokines (Tagawa, 2000; Sprent and Surh, 2003; Abbass and Lichtman, 2006). These are small protein hormones that can stimulate or inhibit many normal cell functions but are less specific and more localized than endocrine hormones (Table 8.2). Cytokines can be divided into several families, including interleukins, interferons, tumour necrosis factors, colony stimulating factors and chemokines, which regulate the migration of cells between and within tissues. For example, there are around 22 different interleukins (ILs), numbered IL-1 to IL-22. Of these, IL-1 is secreted by macrophages and monocytes and can stimulate an inflammatory response and activate lymphocytes (Table 8.2 and Figure 8.2). IL-2 is produced by T-helper lymphocytes and stimulates the proliferation of T-helper cells, cytotoxic T-cells and B-lymphocytes, and activates NK cells. On the other hand, IL-10 and transforming growth factor-β (TGFβ) are immunosuppressants and inhibit the cytotoxic response of the immune system (T-cells and macrophages) against the antigens from tumours and infectious agents (Table 8.2; Levings et al., 2002; Rabson, Roitt and Delves, 2005). Therefore, drugs that block the immunosuppressive action of IL-10 and TGF on the immune system may play an important role in the treatment of human cancers, while those that stimulate their function are useful in suppressing pathological immune responses such as those in autoimmune diseases, allergies and transplantation rejection.

Some of the cytokines are listed in Table 8.2 along with their functions.

ADAPTIVE (ACQUIRED, SPECIFIC) IMMUNE RESPONSE

In many situations, the non-specific immune responses described above (phagocytosis, natural killer cell activation, inflammation), which we are born with and occur in the first few hours of infection, may be sufficient in overcoming the pathogens. If not, disease can ensue and the body must recover by the activation of adaptive immune responses against the invading pathogens (Figure 8.1). There are two types of adaptive immune response, namely AMI and CMI.

The most important cells in providing adaptive immune responses are lymphocytes, which make up between 25% and 35% of white blood cells; their total number in a healthy individual is close to one billion (10^{12}) (Marieb and Hoehn, 2007). Two major types of lymphocyte, called B-cells and T-cells, are present in the blood in a 1:5 ratio. B-cells develop into mature immunocompetent cells in the red bone marrow and each B-cell expresses an antigen receptor (i.e. antibody) of a single specificity on its cell surface. B-cells are responsible for the antibody-mediated immune response (Figure 8.2). In antibody-mediated immunity, the binding of antigen to antigen receptor (i.e. antibody) on B-cells can result in the activation and differentiation of B-cells into antibody-secreting plasma cells. However, ensuring full activation and differentiation of B-cells into plasma cells in response to most antigens, and the antibody class switching (e.g. from low affinity IgM subclass into high affinity IgG subclass), requires a co-stimulator signal, provided by the interaction of B-cells with CD4+ helper T-cells (i.e. T-cells expressing CD4 antigen, see below) (Rabson, Roitt and Delves, 2005).

The binding of CD154 molecules on the CD4+ T-cell to CD40 molecules on the B-cell, together with production of cytokines such as IL-4 and IL-5 by CD4+ helper T-cells, can result in the full activation of B-cells and their differentiation into antibody-producing plasma cells (Figure 8.2) (Abbass and Lichtman, 2006). Each plasma cell then secretes up to 2000 antibodies per second against the original antigen and this process can continue for about 4–5 days. The antibody production by plasma cells can be increased by cytokine IL-6. The secreted antibodies then circulate in the blood and lymphatic system, and bind to the original antigens, marking them for elimination by several mechanisms, including activation of the complement system, promotion of phagocytosis via opsonization and mediation of ADCC with effector cells such as macrophages, NK cells and neutrophils (Figure 8.2).

In contrast to the AMI, a CMI against invading pathogen is mediated by T-cells. Whereas B-cells complete their maturation in bone marrow, T-lymphocytes develop from pre-T-cells in the bone marrow and mature in the thymus into CD4+ or CD8+ expressing T-cells (Figure 8.2). In CMI, CD8+ T-cells, which recognize the target antigen, proliferate and differentiate into CD8+ cytotoxic T-cells (T_c), which kill the target antigens by delivering a lethal dose of the cytokines lymphotoxin and perforin or by directing apoptosis (Figure 8.2) (Marieb and Hoehn, 2007). T-cells expressing CD4+ antigen are called helper T-cells (T_H0) and the binding of antigens to such cells results in their proliferation and differentiation into two CD4+ helper T-cell subsets, T_H1 and T_H2. The T_H1-cells produce cytokines such as IL-2 and IFNγ, which stimulate cell-mediated immune responses against intracellular pathogens and tumour cells. In contrast, T_H2-cells produce cytokines IL-4, IL-5 and IL-6, which play a central role in regulating the antibody-mediated immune response against extracellular antigens and pathogens (Figure 8.2) (Rabson, Roitt and Delves, 2005). The production of cytokines by T_H1-cells can further help the elimination of the target antigen by macrophages of the innate immune system (Figure 8.2). For this reason, CD4+ helper T-cells are viewed as the backbone of the immune system. Their crucial role has been highlighted in patients with AIDS, where the helper T-cells are targeted by the virus (Altfeld and Rosenberg, 2000). In a normal uninfected individual, the number of CD4+ T-cells is between 800 and 1200 cells per cubic millimetre of blood. When the number of CD4+ T-cells falls below 200/mm^3 of blood towards the final stage of HIV infection, patients become particularly susceptible to opportunistic infections by microbes that do not usually cause disease in healthy individuals, as well as to cancers such as Kaposi's sarcoma and lymphomas. Indeed, AIDS cases are part of the evidence supporting both the idea that immunosuppression can increase the incidence of cancer, and the immune surveillance concept (Scadden, 2003; and see below).

In addition to CD8+ cytotoxic T-cells and CD4+ helper T-cells, there are other populations of T-lymphocytes, which inhibit the immune response by releasing inhibitor cytokines. These cells are called suppressor T-cells (T_s) (McHugh and Shevach, 2002; Marieb and Hoehn, 2007).

MHC Molecules and Antigen Recognition and Processing in Cell-Mediated Immunity

As described above, T-lymphocytes are responsible for cell-mediated immunity against foreign antigens. The aim of the majority of cancer vaccines under investigation is to develop antigen-specific T-cell-mediated immune responses against tumour antigens.

However, as with B-cells, successful activation of different T-cells requires the presence of two signals, namely a recognition signal and a co-stimulatory signal. The first signal is recognition of the antigen by the antigen receptors on the surface of the T-cells, called T-cell receptors (TCR), which results in the movement of the T-cells from a resting phase of the cell cycle (G_0) to G_1 phase. However, unlike some B-cells, which can bind directly to an antigen with their unique antigen receptors (i.e. antibodies), the TCRs on both CD4+ and CD8+ T-cells can only recognize a fragment of an antigen that has been processed and presented in association with a unique cell surface self-antigen, called the major histocompatibility complex (MHC) antigen (Rabson, Roitt and Delves, 2005). There are two major types of self-MHC molecule, which are also called human leukocyte antigens (HLAs). MHC class I molecules are found on all body cells except red blood cells, and present the intracellular antigens to the TCRs on CD8+ T-cells. In contrast, class II MHC molecules are present only on the surface of antigen-presenting cells (APCs) such as macrophages, B-lymphocytes and dendritic cells, and are important in the presentation of exogenous antigens to the T-cell receptors on CD4+ helper T-cells (Figure 8.3).

Following the binding of the MHC-antigen fragment complex to the TCR, the T-cells become activated only if they receive a second signal, called a co-stimulatory signal. This second signal has been shown to be essential for full activation of T-cells. The majority of co-stimulatory molecules are cell adhesion molecules, which allow the two cells to adhere to one another for a longer period and result in sustained proliferation and differentiation of T-cells (Figure 8.3). For example, activation and differentiation of CD4+ T-cells into helper T-cells requires the binding of CD28 molecules on CD4+ T-cells to CD80/CD86 molecules present on antigen-presenting cells. This in turn results in the production of IL-2, IL-2 receptor expression and cell cycle progression and proliferation of activated T-cells. In contrast to CD4+ helper T-cells, the full activation of cytotoxic T-cells against the target cells is promoted by the binding of the CD2 molecule on CD8+ T-cells to the CD58 molecule on target cells, and by the interaction of lymphocyte functional antigen-1 (LFA-1) on the T-cell with intercellular adhesion molecule-1 (ICAM-1) on the target cells. Recognition of the antigens by the antigen receptors on the lymphocyte in the absence of co-stimulatory signals results in the production of no cytokines, a state of immunological unresponsiveness called anergy, or even in increased programmed cell death (Frauwirth and Thompson, 2002; Rabson, Roitt and Delves, 2005). Indeed, deficiencies or abnormalities in some of these components can help tumours cells to escape recognition and destruction by T-cells (see below).

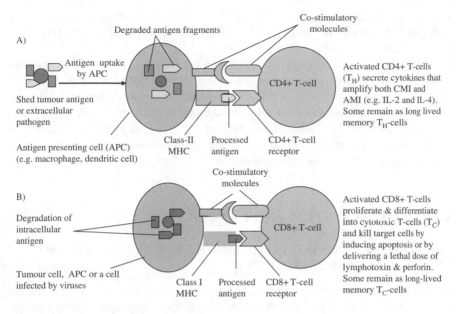

Figure 8.3 Successful activation of antigen-specific T-cell responses requires two signals. (A) CD4+ helper T-cells are only activated when the T-cell receptor recognizes an antigen fragment, from exogenous antigens, in association with class II MHC molecule (signal 1), and receives a co-stimulatory signal by binding the CD28 molecule on T-cells to the CD80/CD86 molecule on the antigen-presenting cell (signal 2). (B) CD8+ T-cells are only activated when the T-cell receptor recognizes an antigen fragment, from endogenous antigens, in association with class I MHC molecule (signal 1), and receives a co-stimulatory signal via interaction between other cell surface (adhesion) molecules (signal 2). Recognition without the second signal results in anergy (a prolonged state of inactivity) and programmed cell death.

Adaptive Immune System, Immunological Memory and Vaccination

Two characteristic features of the adaptive immune response are specificity for a particular antigen and immunological memory. Once the invading pathogens are destroyed by the adaptive immune response, some of the activated B-lymphocytes and T-lymphocytes differentiate into thousands of memory B-cells and memory T-cells. When the body encounters the same pathogen for a second time, these memory cells, which can remain in circulation decades after the first exposure, increase their population so rapidly that the pathogens are destroyed before the body develops any signs of disease (Sprent, 2003; Marieb and Hoehn, 2007).

The development of memory B-cells and memory T-cells against the antigen on the infectious agent or cancer cell is the rationale for successful immunization by vaccination (Wood, 2006). The vaccination of children against infectious agents is estimated to save the lives of 3 million children a year, by helping the body to prevent primary infection (Andre, 2003). The development of vaccines against cancer is more challenging as, unlike vaccines against infectious diseases, cancer vaccines are developed for the treatment of a disease that is already present in the body, and not merely for its prevention (Berd, 1998; Moingeon, 2001; Davidson, Kitchener and Stern, 2002).

In summary, the full activation of the immune system and successful destruction of any foreign antigens, cells and infectious agents by adaptive immune responses requires cooperation between immune cells of adaptive and innate immunity, the production of cytokines by such cells and the presence of co-stimulatory signals, which are essential for activation and proliferation of antigen-specific B-cells and T-cells. Abnormalities in any one of the above components can lead to a state of immunological unresponsiveness against the target antigen.

THE IMMUNE SYSTEM AND CANCER

THE INTERRELATIONSHIP OF IMMUNE RESPONSE, OLD AGE AND HIGH INCIDENCE OF CANCER

In recent years, several factors have been associated with the development of human cancers including smoking, alcohol, diet, air pollution, infectious agents (viruses and bacteria), chemicals, radiation and hereditary factors (see Chapter 2). The treatment of normal cells with these factors results in the mutation of a wide range of genes, such as tumour suppressor genes or genes coding for growth factor, growth factor receptors, motility and invasion factors. Such mutation can result in turn in malignant transformation of normal cells via the expression or release of either abnormal products or a high level of normal products (Hanahan and Weinberg, 2000).

Since the incidence of cancer increases rapidly in old age, ageing is another important factor associated with human cancers. Around 65% of all cancers are diagnosed in people over the age of 65 (see Chapter 2). While the increasing accumulation of mutations in genes over time is one factor contributing to the high incidence of cancers in old age, recent evidence suggests that malfunction of the immune system may also contribute (Ginaldi *et al.*, 2001; Burns and Leventhal, 2000; Effros, 2003). It is well established that with increasing age there is deterioration of the immune response (i.e. immunosenescence), which results in increased susceptibility to infection, insufficient responses to vaccines and a high level of autoimmune disorders (Lords *et al.*, 2001; Stacy *et al.*, 2002; Burns, 2004). In particular, one of the common alterations in old age is a decline in T-cell mediated immune responses. The decline in CMI with age is a multifactorial phenomenon and could be due to: (i) a decrease in the population of naive (resting) T-lymphocytes, with a concomitant increase in the population of antigen-specific memory T-cells (i.e. exhaustion of immune resources); (ii) the poor proliferative response of T-cells to mitogens; and (iii) a decrease in the expression of the co-stimulatory molecule (e.g. CD28) on T-cells, together with an increase in the expression of inhibitory molecule on CD4+ helper T-cells (Franceschi, Bonafe and Valensin, 2000; Appay and Rowland-Jones, 2002; Effros, 2003). While there is no significant change in the antibody-mediated immune responses and the innate immune response is largely unchanged or even up-regulated in old age, a decline in the T-cell-mediated immune responses, such as those mediated by CD4+ helper T-cells (Figure 8.2), can reduce the overall immune response against cancer cells (Miller, 1996; Lords *et al.*, 2001; Chen, Flurkey and Harrison, 2002; Kovaiou and Grubeck-Loebenstein, 2006).

THE IMMUNE SURVEILLANCE THEORY

The immune surveillance theory put forward by Thomas in 1959 and redefined by Burnett states that the immune system is constantly patrolling the body for tumour (abnormal) cells, which are recognized as foreign, and that when they are found it mounts an immune response that results in their elimination before they become clinically detectable (Burnet, 1967). Although this concept remains controversial, a wide range of evidence supports the idea.

First, cancer patients with tumours infiltrated by many immune cells (e.g. proliferating CD8+ T-lymphocytes, macrophages, NK cells) have a better survival rate than those with few infiltrated immune cells, suggesting that such immune cells are responsible for the improved survival in these patients (Ropponen *et al.*, 1997; Naito *et al.*, 1998; Nakano *et al.*, 2001; Nakayama *et al.*, 2002; Ohno *et al.*, 2002). Second, as described above, the incidence of cancer is higher in older people and in the neonatal period, when immune responses are less efficient. Third, the incidence of cancer is much higher in immunodeficient people (e.g. AIDS patients), than those with a normal immune system. About 40% of HIV infected individuals develop some form of cancer, such as Kaposi's sarcoma, a malignant tumour of the blood vessels in the skin, or lymphoma, a malignant tumour of the lymphatic system (Scadden, 2003). In addition, the incidence of certain types of cancer (e.g. skin cancers, lymphoma) is increased by 400−500-fold in patients with organ transplants, whose immune systems have been down-regulated with immunosuppressive drugs, and reversing the immunosuppression can result in tumour regression (Abgrall *et al.*, 2002; Lutz and Heemann, 2003; Vial and Descotes, 2003). Furthermore, spontaneous regression of malignant tumours occurs in patients with melanoma, renal cell carcinoma, neuroblastoma, lymphoma and hepatocellular carcinoma, in which the immune system plays an important role (Papac, 1998; Bromberg, Siemers and Taphoorn, 2002; Morimoto *et al.*, 2002).

MECHANISMS RESPONSIBLE FOR TUMOURS ESCAPING IMMUNE RECOGNITION

The proliferation and presence of clinically detectable tumours in cancer patients suggests that such tumours have been able to escape recognition and destruction by the immune system (i.e. the immune surveillance). From examination of sera and biopsies from cancer patients, it has become evident that cancer patients can produce both cell-mediated and antibody-mediated immune responses against tumour cells (Naito *et al.*, 1998; Shimada, Ochiai and Nomura, 2003). However, recent evidence suggests that the immune responses in some patients are either too weak to be effective in eliminating all tumours or, in other cases, only able to recognize the original tumours. Indeed, as explained in Chapter 10, the great majority of human tumour antigens are tumour-associated antigens, and such antigens are also present in lower amounts on normal cells and are therefore less immunogenic (Kuroki *et al.*, 2002). Several other factors have been identified that can help the tumour cells to escape recognition and destruction by the immune system (Table 8.4). In some situations, tumour cells escape immune recognition by losing or down-regulating the expression of highly immunogenic antigens (Lollini and Forni, 2003). In other cases, tumour cells have been shown to lose or down-regulate the expression of class-I MHC molecules, which are essential (Figure 8.2) for antigen recognition and cell killing by CD8+ cytotoxic T-cells (Natali *et al.*, 1989; Paschen *et al.*, 2003). Antigen presentation by antigen-presenting cells to T-cells in the absence of a co-stimulatory signal or mitogenic cytokines (e.g. IL-2) can result in immunological anergy. The release of immunosuppressive cytokines such as TGFβ and IL-10 by tumour cells and T-cells can suppress the immune response against cancer cells, leading to tumour tolerance (Kirkbride and Blobe, 2003; Rabson, Roitt and Delves, 2005).

IMMUNOTHERAPEUTIC STRATEGIES FOR HUMAN CANCER

In recent years, due to better understanding of the immune system, including the mechanisms that are used by tumour cells to escape immune recognition and destruction, and identification of novel antigens of biological and clinical significance at different stages of cancer, immunotherapeutic approaches have been initiated in patients with a wide range of cancers (Berd, 1998; Armstrong and Hawkins, 2001; Costello *et al.*, 2003; Waldman, 2003). The overall aim of such strategies is to provide protection against cancer cells, either by amplifying the immune response against cancer cells or by correcting and breaking tolerance against tumour antigens using the patient's own immune system.

There are currently two main immunotherapeutic strategies against human cancers, namely: the monoclonal antibody-based therapy of human cancer and

Table 8.4 Factors which may help tumour cells to escape immune recognition

- Loss or down-regulation of antigens recognized by tumour cells.
- Down-regulation of class-I MHC expression from the tumour cell's surface.
- Lack of co-stimulatory molecules (e.g. cytokines and adhesion molecules) which are necessary for T-cell activation.
- Overwhelming mass of tumour antigens and the presence of shed antigens in circulation.
- Increased level of immunosuppressive cytokines (TGFß or IL-10).
- Down-regulation of antigen processing machinery.

the development of cancer vaccines. The former strategy is described in detail in Chapter 10, and is particularly effective in the destruction of extracellular antigens, such as overexpressed HER-2 antigens, in patients with breast cancer.

In recent years, several types of cancer vaccine have been prepared, including vaccines containing: (i) intact autologous tumour cells (derived from the patient to be treated) or intact allogeneic tumour cells (derived from other patients), modified by physical alteration, gene modification (with IL-2, GM-CSF) or mixing with adjuvants (e.g. BCG, an attenuated strain of *Mycobacterium bovis,* or QS-21, a material extracted from tree bark) which boost the immune response against human tumour cells; (ii) crude extracts of tumour cells; (iii) purified extracts (e.g. gangliosides in melanoma); (iv) peptides (MAGE proteins found in melanoma); (v) heat-shock proteins; (vi) dendritic cells pulsed with tumour antigens and co-stimulatory molecules and cytokines; (vii) DNA and RNA-based vaccines; and (viii) anti-idiotypic antibodies as surrogate antigens (Pardoll, 1998; Leitner, Ying and Restifo, 2000; Berd, 2001; Lundqvist and Pisa, 2002; Davidson, Kitchener and Stern, 2002; Ehrke, 2003). The major aim of such vaccines is to direct tumour killing by inducing cell mediated (antigen-specific T-cell) anti-tumour immune responses in patients. The extraordinary capacity of dendritic cells for capturing and processing tumour antigens, together with their capacity to present the fragments of such antigens, in association with MHC class I and MHC class II molecules, to CD4+ T-cells and CD8+ T-cells, leading to their activation, have made them ideal as sources of human cancer vaccines (Figure 8.4; Buchsel and DeMeyer, 2006).

In June 2006, the Food and Drug Administration (United States) approved the use of a vaccine called Gardasil against human papillomavirus (HPV), to protect women against cervical cancer, precancerous lesions and genital warts. Cervical cancer is the second most common cancer in women and kills more than 288 000 worldwide each year. More than 95% of invasive cervical cancer is caused by human HPVs (McLemore, 2006). Gardasil is developed by Merck & amp; Co. and is effective against HPV types 16 and 18, which cause more than two-thirds of cervical cancer, and HPV types 6 and 11, which are responsible for 90% of genital warts. Gardasil is a recombinant quadrivalent vaccine containing a mixture of the viral-like particles derived from the L1 capsid proteins of HPV-6, HPV-11, HPV-16 and HPV-18, and an aluminium-containing adjuvant. The results of four clinical trials conducted in 21 000 women and teenage girls have shown that Gardasil is nearly 100% effective in preventing precancerous cervical, vaginal, vulvar and genital lesions caused by HPV-16 and HPV-18, and 99% effective in preventing genital warts caused by HPV-6 and HPV-11. Gardasil was approved by the FDA for girls or women aged 9 to 26, and is given as three injections over a six-month period (Widdice and Kahn, 2006). A second HPV vaccine called Cervarix is in the final stages of development by GlaxoSmithKline and encouraging results have been reported with this bivalent (HPV-16 and HPV-18) vaccine (Speck and Tyring, 2006). GlaxoSmithKline filed Cervarix for approval with the European Union regulators in September 2006. It is expected to be approved in the United States and other countries in early 2007.

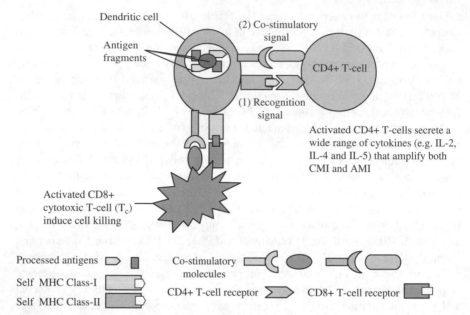

Figure 8.4 Therapeutic strategy using dendritic cells as a source of cancer vaccine. Dendritic cells express high levels of both class I MHC and class II MHC molecules on their cell surface. They can be harvested from cancer patients, loaded with human tumour antigens, pulsed with co-stimulatory molecules and returned to patients. Such cells can then present the tumour antigen fragments, in association with class I MHC, to cytotoxic CD8+ T-cells and therefore mediate tumour cell killing by CMI. In addition, some of the antigen processed by dendritic cells can be presented in association with class II MHC molecules to CD4+ helper T-cells, which secrete a wide range of cytokines that help cell killing via CMI and AMI and activate macrophage cell killing (see Figure 8.2).

Unlike Gardasil, Cervarix does not protect against HPV-6 and HPV-11 and therefore will not prevent genital warts. The HPV vaccines are highly immunogenic, provide protection by generating anti-HPV antibodies and have the potential for reducing the incidence of cervical cancer by 70% (Widdice and Kahn, 2006). The results of ongoing clinical trials with different types of vaccine should clarify the full potential and limitation of each strategy and could ultimately lead to the development of an effective therapeutic strategy directed against a specific population of cancer patients (Tjoa *et al.*, 1997; Bremers *et al.*, 2000; Bodey *et al.*, 2000; Romero *et al.*, 2002; Sabel and Sondak, 2002; Boon and Van den Enbde, 2003; Ehrke, 2003; Girard, Osmoanove and Kieny, 2006; Widdice and Kahn, 2006).

IMMUNE SYSTEM IN PATIENTS UNDERGOING CHEMOTHERAPY AND RADIOTHERAPY

All the immune cells of our body (e.g. neutrophils, lymphocytes, monocytes, NK cells) are developed from stem cells in the bone marrow. In the bone marrow, there is approximately 1 stem cell for every 100 000 blood cells. Neutrophils account for about 54−63% of all white blood cells and are the first immune cells to arrive at the site of infection and the first line of defence against invading pathogens. Their numbers in circulation do not change with age in normal individuals (see above). Since they have a short half-life in the blood, the bone marrow produces about 10^{11} neutrophils a day. Lymphocytes are also very important in mediating adaptive immune responses against both intracellular and extracellular antigens and cancer cells. About one thousand million lymphocytes die and are replaced by the stem cells in the bone marrow every day.

One of the common and most dangerous side effects associated with an intensive course of chemotherapy and radiotherapy is bone marrow suppression and a consequent reduction in the number of white blood cells (leucocytes) in the blood, a condition called leucopenia (Kubota et al., 2001; Hood, 2003). In particular, febrile neutropenia is a common complication of cancer chemotherapy which can cause death in 4−21% of cancer patients (Young and Feld, 2000; Ray-Coquard et al., 2003). With advances in genetic engineering, recombinant forms of haematopoietic cytokines, also called colony stimulating factor (CSF), have been generated which stimulate the proliferation and differentiation of different populations of white blood cells. For example, the human granulocyte colony stimulating factor filgrastim has been shown to be effective in reducing neutropenia, decreasing its severity and duration, reducing hospitalizations and the incidence of infection, and improving quality of life in patients undergoing chemotherapy (Valley, 2002). A modified version of filgrastim, called pegfilgrastim, has been developed which has a much longer serum half-life and therefore requires less frequent administration (Crawford, 2002; Hood, 2003; Rader, 2006).

CONCLUSION

A better understanding of our immune system and the way it can differentiate between self-antigens and non-self-antigens will have a huge impact on various areas of clinical medicine. Such developments could help treatment of patients with cancer, infection, autoimmune diseases, allergies, as well those undergoing organ transplants or requiring aggressive forms of chemotherapy or radiotherapy.

In relation to cancer, it is clear that with the identification of novel antigens that not only play a crucial role in the biology and pathology of different types of cancer but also activate both cell-mediated and antibody-mediated immune response, a more effective immunotherapeutic strategy for educating our immune system (i.e. cancer vaccines) could be developed. In this way, persistent tumour antigens would be recognized and remembered by the memory B-cells and T-cells already present in the immune system, leading to the prevention of the majority of human cancers. However, as discussed above, vaccination against such persistent tumour antigens should be performed in the young, while their immune system is most efficient in recognizing and destroying foreign antigens. Recent advances in tumour immunology, cell and molecular biology of cancer, together with technological advances in genetic engineering and development of monoclonal antibodies (Chapter 10), makes the routine use of immunological approaches for the prevention and treatment of human cancers imminent.

9 Tumour Markers

If a clinician was asked to name a tumour marker, they would invariably name one of the commonly tested serum tumour markers that they use in their clinical management to monitor patients with cancer who have undergone treatment and are in the remission. The named ones would include: carcinoembryonic antigen (CEA), cancer antigen 125 (CA125), cancer antigen 15-3 (CA15-3), carbohydrate antigen 19-9 (CA19-9), β human chorionic gonadotrophin (β-hCG), α-fetoprotein (AFP), lactic acid dehydrogenase (LDH), thyroglobulin and prostate specific antigen (PSA). The tumour markers' names give an indication of the diversity of the biological structural groups they cover: carbohydrates, hormones, enzymes, proteins and immunoglobulins.

WHAT ARE TUMOUR MARKERS?

The National Cancer Institute (NCI) *Dictionary of Cancer Terms* provides a simple definition of a tumour marker, similar to that used by many others: 'a substance that is sometimes found in the blood, other body fluids, or tissues. A high level of tumour marker may mean that a certain type of cancer is in the body. Also called biomarkers.'

However, since 1988 the accepted, more comprehensive definition of a tumour marker has been:

> Biochemical tumor marker are substances developed in tumor cells and secreted into body fluids in which they can be quantitated by non-invasive analyses. Because of a correlation between marker concentration and active tumor mass, tumor markers are useful in the management of cancer patients. Markers, which are available for most cancer cases, are additional, valuable tools in patient prognosis, surveillance and therapy monitoring, whereas

The Biology of Cancer, Second Edition. Edited by J. Gabriel
© 2007 John Wiley & Sons, Ltd.

they are presently not applicable for screening. Serodiagnostic measurements of markers should emphasize relative trends instead of absolute values and cut-off levels.

Suresh (2001), The Fifth International Conference on Human Tumour Markers held in Stockholm, Sweden in 1988

In essence, both definitions are predominately describing serum tumour markers, which are the most frequently used in monitoring the effectiveness of cancer therapy as part of the clinical management of patients undergoing treatment. As blood samples are now a routine part of a patient's care, they provide a convenient and safe method for monitoring tumour markers.

The definitions can now be expanded to include advances in technology that permit measurements of a tumour marker either qualitatively or quantitatively by chemical, immunological, genomic or proteomic methods.

Tumour markers exist as a result of events within a tumour's development that are governed by genetic or epigenetic mechanisms and signalling pathways. These complex intracellular molecular pathways are not yet fully understood, nor is the mechanism by which the tumour cells control and co-opt the neighbouring non-neoplastic cells in the process of tumourigenesis. Often mutation of regulatory oncogenes such as ras, c-myc and p53 and their expressed proteins is found to have increased in the majority of cancer cells. The process of carcinogenesis may be disrupted at any stage, which results in heterogeneity among tumours of the same type and also within the same tumour mass. This is due to a tumour cell's intrinsic genetic instability (Hanahan and Weinberg, 2000).

Tumour tissue is often less differentiated than normal tissue, and histologically it resembles foetal embryonic tissue rather than normal adult tissue. In many cases the tumour markers are embryonic substances that are not expressed by the differentiated normal adult tissue. These biological substances can be attributed to the events in tumourigenesis. They may be produced by the tumour cells themselves, by the body in response to the presence of cancer, or in certain benign conditions, for example dermatofibroma, benign prostatic hyperplasia and benign prostatic hypertrophy. Those substances produced intracellularly, or on the cell membrane (oestrogen receptor − ER) are detected by immunohistochemistry (IHC) on the tumour tissue. Those secreted into body fluids can be quantified by immunoassay methods. The marker's production can be due to:

- Unique genes only expressed in tumour cells (Cancer antigen 125 − CA125).
- Abnormal or higher than normal expressions of specific biochemical substances (prostatic acid phosphate − pap; β_2-microglobulin − β_2M; growth factors; cytokines) found in normal cells.
- Expression of foetal antigens normally expressed during embryological development but not present in normal adult tissue − known as oncofoetal antigens (α-foetal protein − AFP). Hence the fact that the morphology of the cancer tissue on histological examination often resembles foetal tissue rather than normal adult differentiated tissue.

Markers found in normal tissue, or benign conditions, are often referred to as 'tumour-associated antigens'.

As already mentioned, these 'cancer' markers can be divided into two groups:

- Tumour Markers – tumour-specific glycoproteins and mucins expressed only in tumour cells (CA125, CA19-9).
- Tumour-Associated Markers – oncofoetal antigens, oncogenes, oncoproteins, carbohydrates, hormones, enzymes, cytokines, soluble receptors, growth factors, cellular markers – not tumour-specific, but expressed in higher levels than normal tissue (CEA, AFP, β_2M, p21, Ras protein, Vascular endothelial growth factor – VEGF).

Which marker to measure is determined by the tumour type and whether the marker levels are likely to change during the course of the patient's disease. These markers fall into two categories (Fertig and Hayes, 2001):

- Static – tend to remain constant throughout the natural history of a cancer and are measured once. These may be used as a prognostic indicator. They are usually measured by IHC on tissue samples. Examples include ER in breast cancer, HER-2/neu (c-erbB-2) and mutant p53.
- Dynamic – reflect the activity of the tumour. Levels may respond to changes in the tumour due to therapy, and may be useful to predict response. These are normally measured in blood and body fluids. Examples include CA125 and CA19-9.

To date, no tumour marker has yet been found to be specific and sufficiently sensitive enough to be the sole indicator of cancer or to be of use in mass screening programmes (Suresh, 2001; Schilsky and Taube, 2002; Duffy and McGing, 2005).

The limitations of tumour markers are:

- Must be used in conjunction with other investigative procedures, for example CT imaging.
- Functional biological substances produced by normal tissues and only potentially elevated in tumour cells.
- Most are not tissue- or tumour-specific but are found with different tumours of the same tissue type (tumour-associated antigens).
- They are usually elevated at later stages of cancer disease, therefore not sensitive enough for use as a screening diagnostic test for early-stage disease.
- They may be elevated in other non-cancerous diseases, for example benign and inflammatory.
- With a few exceptions such as ER, progesterone receptor (PR) or HER2/neu (c-erbB-2), most tumour markers cannot be used to predict therapeutic response to treatment and enable the patient to benefit from individualized therapy.
- Tumour marker levels are not altered in all people with cancer, especially if the cancer is at an early stage.

The first tumour marker to be associated with a tumour was Bence Jones protein (BJP). It was identified in 1846 from the acidified urine of some patients with cancer, and over 150 years later is still used as a tumour marker for myeloma. It has been identified as consisting of monoclonal free light chains of immunoglobulins. BJP concentrations are found to be raised in more than 50% of patients with multiple myeloma (Kyle, 1975; Magdelenat, 1992; Thomas and Sweep, 2001).

Since 1846, other proteins, enzymes, isoenzymes, receptors, structural elements and hormones have been associated with various tumour types to be used as tumour markers, biomarkers or cancer markers in blood and other body fluids (ascites, faecal occult blood, etc.) for patients with growing tumours. Examples include acid phosphatase for prostate cancer, α- fetoprotein (AFP) for hepatoma and carcinoembryonic antigen (CEA) for colorectal cancer. However, it was not until the early 1960s that trace amounts of these secreted tumour markers were measurable from body fluids by radioimmunoassay (RIA) methods (Yalow and Berson, 1960; Miles and Hales, 1968). Further advances in immunoassay technologies in the 1970s and 1980s, in particular the use of monoclonal antibodies (Köhler and Milstein, 1975), have helped identify many new tumour markers. The use of recombinant DNA and non-radioactive detection methods has led to the development of automated immunoassay systems.

It has only been since the mid-1990s, following detailed analysis of all the published literature relating to tumour markers (including clinical trials) by various panels of experts at international, national and regional levels, that tumour markers have been fully validated for clinical use within evidence-based medicine. The findings of these multidisciplinary expert panels have been published as recommendations and guidelines. Examples include:

• Tumor Marker Expert Panel, American Society of Clinical Oncology (ASCO). Clinical practice guidelines for the use of tumor markers in breast and colorectal cancer. 1996.
• European Group for Tumor Markers (EGTM): Consensus recommendations. 1999.
• 2000 update of recommendations for the use of tumor markers in breast and colorectal cancer: clinical practice guidelines of the American Society of Clinical Oncology (ASCO). 2001.
• European Society for Medical Oncology (ESMO). ESMO minimum clinical recommendations for diagnosis, treatment and follow-up of ovarian cancer. 2001.
• Clinical utility of biochemical markers in colorectal cancer: European Group on Tumor Markers (EGTM) guidelines. 2003.
• Association of Clinical Biochemists in Ireland. Guidelines for the use of tumor markers. 2005.
• ASCO 2006 Update of Recommendations for the Use of Tumor Markers in Gastrointestinal Cancer. 2006.

These guidelines have a tendency either to favour clinical aspects of care (e.g. surgery) or to focus on laboratory investigations for monitoring a patient's disease through the measurement of tumour markers (Sturgeon, 2002). These recommendations and guidelines have resulted in only a handful of serum tumour markers being recommended for clinical use. Others are still being investigated in ongoing clinical trials. However, these guidelines can vary in their recommendations (Sturgeon, 2002); it is advisable to consult your hospital local guidelines.

Today, with the development of automated immunoassays, tumour markers can be routinely measured in clinical biochemistry laboratories rather than in specialist laboratories. They are commonly used in the clinical management of a patient, giving an indication that the patient's tumour is not responding to treatment, or has metastasized and warrants further investigation.

In establishing a cancer diagnosis, only a limited number of markers can be used at initial diagnosis, in conjunction with other investigations, to assist in staging and grading of the tumour and in prognosis, such as oestrogen receptor, progesterone and HER-2/neu. The majority of other markers cannot be used due to low sensitivity, and lack of specificity during the early stages of a patient's disease. However, establishing the initial baseline level of an appropriate tumour marker at the time of diagnosis is vital and essential if tumour markers are to be used as a non-invasive method for monitoring a patient's response to treatment, even though the results may not contribute to the diagnosis. Often clinicians overlook a request for a tumour marker test at the pre-treatment stage, but this is where care pathways play a crucial role in equity of management. A decrease in the marker level may be an indication that the cancer has responded favourably to therapy. In the case of post-surgery or radiotherapy, this would suggest that treatment has been successful. Conversely, if levels remain constant, or indeed rise, it may be an indication that the tumour is not responding to treatment, signalling recurrence or a metastasis of the tumour (Bidart et al., 1999). A rise in a tumour marker's level may be used as an early warning sign and can precede confirmation of the presence of a tumour by imaging investigations by up to several months.

Once a patient's tumour markers are measured by one laboratory, that laboratory should be used for testing all subsequent serial/longitudinal samples from the patient to maintain consistency, that is to ensure the same assay methodology of the same manufacture is being used. Different values may be obtained between laboratories, even between those using automated systems, as can be seen from analysis of the results from an external quality control assurance scheme (Sturgeon and Seth, 1996; Sturgeon et al., 1999b) (Table 9.1).

LABORATORY ASPECTS

ASSAY TECHNOLOGY

Tumour markers are predominately measured by immunochemistry techniques (IHC, FISH) and immunoassays. A number of different assay formats are used, depending on the technology platform employed. Most immunoassays for tumour markers now mainly use the 2-site immunometric (sandwich) immunoassay format;

Table 9.1   Examples of some of the most frequently requested tumour markers and their associated cancers

Tumour Marker		Associated Tumour
AFP	α1-fetoprotein	Liver, germ cell (testis and ovary). Used together with β-hCG.
β-2M	Beta-2-microglobulin	B-cell lymphoma multiple myeloma, chronic lymphocytic leukaemia
β-hCG	β-human chorionic gonadotrophin	Choriocarcinoma, germ cell (testis and ovary). Used together with AFP
CA15-3	Cancer antigen 15-3	Metastatic breast cancer and adenocarcinomas. Alternative to CA 27.29
CA 27.29	Cancer antigen 27.29	Metastatic breast cancer and adenocarcinomas. Alternative to CA15-3
CA19-9	Carbohydrate antigen 19-9	Pancreatic, gastric and colon cancer
CA125	Cancer antigen 125	Epithelial ovarian cancer, advanced adenocarcinoma
CEA	Carcinoembryonic antigen	Advanced adenocarcinomas, other GI tract cancer, breast, liver and lung
LDH	Lactic acid Dehydrogenase Isoenzyme 5	Germ cell tumours
PSA	Prostate-specific antigen	Prostate cancer. Separate assays used for free and total PSA

use of this format depends on the available epitopes presence on the antigen concerned. The assay format often employs a matched pair of monoclonal anti-bodies, or a monoclonal and a polyclonal antibody specific for the marker concerned. One is used as a capture antibody bound to the solid phase, while the other is used as a labelled detection antibody. The patient's sample is incubated in the captured antibody solid phase; any specific antigen in the sample is then bound to the anti-body, with unbound material being removed by washing. The detection antibody is added, and binds to any captured antigen. Unbound detection antibody is removed by washing, and the bound detection antibody is measured. An alternative to the sequential assay approach is a simultaneous immunometric immunoasay format, where the detection antibody can be incubated at the same time as the patient's sample.

Another format often employed is the competitive immunoassay. As an example, in the case CA27.29, where there is a single epitope, recombinant CA27.29 antigen is bound to the solid phase. The patient's sample is then incubated in the solid phase in the presence of labelled detection antibody. Antigen in the patient's sample competes with the antigen bound on the solid phase for the labelled antibody. Any detection antibody that has bound to the antigen in the sample and not bound to the solid-phase antigen is removed by washing. The presence of labelled detection antibody is then measured. Reduction in the labelled detection antibody signal is an indication that the detection antibody has bound to the antigen in the patient's sample. Absence of antigen in the patient's sample would be indicated by high detection antibody signal, that is, detection antibody binding to the antigen on the solid phase.

A number of different technologies are used, employing different detection systems. For ^{125}I radiolabel antibody (radioimmunoassay — RIAs), a gamma counter is used to measure the gamma emissions; for colorimetric enzymes system (Enzyme-Linked Immunosorbent Assay — ELISA or EIA), the absorbance of the colour change of precipitating substrate in the presence of the enzyme-labelled antibody is measured spectrometrically; for luminescence systems, light-emitting substrates in the presence of enzyme-labelled antibody are measured, either by luminometer or by time-resolved imaging with charged coupled devices (CCD) camera; for fluorescence using fluorescein or fluorophore-labelled antibody, emission of fluorescence at specific wavelengths is detected by photodetector/CDD camera after excitation at another wavelength from polarized light or a laser (Figure 9.1).

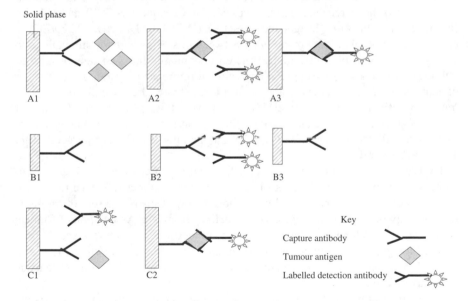

Figure 9.1 Immunometric sandwich assay. The various stages of two sandwich assay formats are shown. A1–A3: sequential; and C1–C2: simultaneous. A1: sample incubated on the solid phase, coated with capture antibody for a specific tumour antigen; A2: after washing to remove any unbound antigen, labelled detection antibody for specific antigen is added to the solid phase and incubated; A3: after washing any labelled detection antibody that has bound to antigen/capture antibody complex is detected. B1–B3 shows the results of an unreactive sample, absence of antigen/capture antibody labelled detection antibody complex.

QUALITY ASSURANCE AND STANDARDIZATION

Quality assurance is fundamental for any diagnostic laboratory performing and reporting assay results to clinicians. Being aware of the limitations of the assay should avoid any adverse effect on patient treatment.

One of the problems with tumour marker assays in the past has been the lack of standardization, in that one assay may not be comparable to another for a particular marker. One antibody derived against a particular antigen can have a different affinity and specificity for an epiotope than another. The assay may recognize only a subunit of the antigen rather than total antigen.

The International Society for Oncodevelopmental Biology and Medicine (ISOBM) is addressing this issue by validating and characterizing the antibodies, and mapping the epitopes to specific antibodies. The monoclonal antibodies are compared and assessed against a particular tumour marker for their suitability as 'capture' or 'detection' antibodies, and for how they perform as a matched pair. This evaluation is usually conducted by comparison of performance of different manufactured assays for a particular assay. The ISOBM has also agreed on the structure of some of the marker antigens (Nustad *et al.,* 1996; Stenman *et al.,* 1999).

These assays now have to meet more stringent regulation requirements on their suitability for diagnostic use worldwide. In the United States, only a few tumour marker assays have received FDA approval, for example CA27.29 and CA125. In Europe, the In Vitro Diagnostic Directive (IVDD − Directive 98/79/EC) is addressing the problem of comparability between kits. Kit standards are required to correspond to available international reference standards for each tumour marker, although many markers lack agreed international reference preparations. A number of manufacturers with assays using similar formats are already collaborating, for mutual benefit, in calibrating their kit standards to this specification. The use of tumour marker reference control sera in these assays is strongly recommended, to assist standardization between laboratories and manufacturers' kits (Sturgeon *et al.,* 1996, 1999b, 2001).

To date, many tumour markers still lack an agreed international reference standard. Another problem is the lack of agreed consensus about reference ranges for tumour markers. These can vary by 10-fold or more. Generally users of the same methodology quote similar ranges. The guidelines from The Association of Clinical Biochemists in Ireland (1999 and 2005) recommend reference ranges should only be used for guidance and suggest trends in changes of levels are clinically useful rather than absolute values. Laboratory reports should reflect this and state the name of the assay used.

The participation in external quality control assessments (proficiency) is assisting standardization of tumour marker testing between laboratories. An EORTC external quality programme for ER and PgR between 1998 and 1999 examined two assays, Ligand Binding Assay (LBA) and Enzyme Immuno Assay (EIA), used by 42 and 39 participants respectively. The initial results showed coefficiency of variation (CV) between laboratories for the two assays to be 40−50%. After normalization of the results, CV values between laboratories dropped to 11% for ER LBA and 14% for

ER EIA. The results demonstrated the need to calibrate assays between laboratories, an essential requirement for data obtained in multicentre clinical studies (Sweep and Geurts-Moespot, 2000).

The European Group for Tumor Markers (EGTM) has recommended that, for most tumour marker assays on automated systems, performance CVs of $<5\%$ (intra-assay) and $<10\%$ (inter-assay) can be achievable.

In the United Kingdom, active participation in the National External Quality Assurance Scheme (NEQAS) is stipulated in the National Cancer Measures (DoH, 2004). An NEQAS participation certificate for each test performed by a laboratory, if that test is included in the scheme, must be provided during peer review and other audits.

In addition, the testing laboratory must ensure good laboratory practice (written protocols for validated assays, frequent equipment calibration, acceptance criteria and monitoring, i.e. Westgard rules, documentation, audit, trials, etc.). The laboratories performing these investigations should be accredited (quality mark) and able to demonstrate their quality system to an audit by external peer reviewers, showing that they meet the accreditation awarding body's exacting standards. In the United Kingdom, the accreditation awarding body for clinical laboratories is the Clinical Pathology Accreditation (CPA) (UK) Limited.

One of the most essential procedures is the use of internal quality control (IQC) samples in every assay. The IQC sample must mimic the patient's samples and must not be from the same manufacture as the assay, that is, independent of the assay manufacture. The use of IQC samples ensures the assay is robust, reproducible and, used with Westgard rules, will highlight any system failure and show whether recalibration is required (Westgard et al., 1981; Westgard and Barry, 1986).

Understanding the limitation of an assay is essential to avoid erroneous results. One such limitation is in sample collection intervals; knowledge of tumour marker half-life and doubling times is important when scheduling sampling time between samples. Bidart and his colleagues suggested:

> the use tumour kinetics rather than cut-off values may often provide the most relevant predictive factors for the estimation of disease-free and overall survival, treatment efficacy, and for the decision regarding optimal treatment and cost-effectiveness in terms of toxicity and patient benefit.
>
> *Bidart et al. (1999)*

Other limiting factors include interference in assays from auto- and heterophilic antibodies in the patient's sample, which can lead to erroneous results (Kricka, 2000; Marks, 2002).

The use of monoclonal antibody therapy has led to another possible source of interference, that is human anti-mouse monoclonal antibodies (HAMA). In the United States, the FDA requires that manufacturers of assays specifically draw attention to HAMA as a potential problem. It is essential that the clinician provide all the relevant clinical information when requesting a tumour marker test; in particular, that any monoclonal therapy a patient may have received is clearly indicated.

The laboratory can then perform the appropriate pre-treatment before the sample is tested for a tumour marker.

Another problem can be an inappropriate sample type. In the case of vascular endothelial growth factor (VEGF) measurements, citrated, EDTA-treated or heparinized plasma are the samples of choice. If serum samples are used, VEGF can be released from platelets and other blood components during blood clotting, leading to increased levels compared to plasma samples (Webb *et al.*, 1998; Adams *et al.*, 2000).

(It is advisable to refer to the local pathology laboratory's testing schedule for a list of the services they offer and their sample requirements for a particular test.)

WHAT ARE THE USES OF TUMOUR MARKERS IN DISEASE MANAGEMENT?

The decision to test for tumour markers can depend on an individual clinician's management plan and/or the patient care pathway. Several guidelines have now been produced by a number of expert panels to provide information regarding patient care. Examples include guidelines by the American Society of Clinical Oncology (ASCO), which recommends that only oestrogen receptor (ER) and progesterone receptor (PR) values are of useful benefit in predicting breast cancer patients suitable for endocrine therapy (ASCO, 1996, 1998; Hammond and Taube, 2002); the College of American Pathologists (CAP), which has evaluated tumour markers, both in 1994 and 1999, has identified those recommended for clinical use for breast, prostate and colon cancer (Henson *et al.*, 1995; Hammond *et al.*, 2000; Hammond and Taube, 2002).

The reviews of the various guidelines from multidisciplinary expert panels at international, national and regional levels have found that, although substantial research has been or is being performed in the field of tumour markers, very little has been done on how this translates into clinical practice (Hayes, Trock and Harris, 1998; Sturgeon, 2002).

Martin Fleisher and his colleagues (2002) have comprehensively reviewed these expert panels' guidelines. The guidelines were based on stringent methodologies and are regularly reviewed and updated to reflect evidence-based publications. In the majority of cases the evidence-based references were cited.

Catharine Sturgeon, one of the authors of the Fleisher review, has written a further outline summary of the review (Sturgeon, 2002). Sturgeon found the guidelines can be categorized into two groups: (i) tumour markers for specific cancers (ASCO) and (ii) tumour markers for a range of cancers (EGTM, ABCI, NACB). Their recommendations are fairly general, providing advice about which markers to measure in specific malignancies and their appropriate application. They were found to focus either on the clinical aspects (surgery, radiotherapy, etc.) or on laboratory investigations. Overall, the guidelines provide valuable consensus documents on the management of specific cancers and need to be referred to when drawing up local protocols. A multidisciplinary team approach, consisting of both clinicians and laboratorians, should be considered when developing local protocols (DoH, 2000b). Sturgeon suggests that consideration should be given to how best to implement, publish, disseminate and promote ownership of the local protocol. Sturgeon recommends the development of audit procedures to monitor the effectiveness of clinical practice.

Useful Markers for Disease Management

The UK guidelines agree that tumour markers (primary due to specificity and sensitivity) should not be used for screening. Otherwise, they are involved in staging and prognosis, detection of recurrence, follow-up and monitoring.

The most common serum tumour markers currently used as surrogates to monitor the course of a disease during and following treatment are: cancer antigen 125 (CA-125) and carbohydrate antigen 19-9 (CA19-9) for ovarian cancer; carcinoembryonic antigen (CEA) for colorectal cancer; prostate-specific antigen (PSA) for prostate cancer; and α-fetoprotein (AFP), beta human chorionic gonadotrophin (β-HCG) and lactic acid dehydrogenase isoenzyme (LDH) for germ cell tumour.

For patients with breast cancer, it is possible to predict who is likely to benefit from endocrine therapy hormone treatment. Suitability for treatment is determined by the presence of oestrogen and progesterone receptors in the cancer tissue. Over 60% of patients whose cancer is receptor positive will respond to treatment, compared to 10% of those whose cancer is receptor negative. Detection of the overexpression of HER-2/neu (c-erb-2) occurs in 20–30% of breast cancer and is a requirement for receiving Herceptin therapy. HER-2/neu levels can identify women who are likely to benefit from trastuzumab (Herceptin) treatment or anthracycline-based treatments (adriamycin, doxorubicin, epirubicin).

Due to the low sensitivity and low specificity of cancer antigen 15-3 (CA 15-3), or BR27.29, it is not recommended that these MUC-1 tumour markers are used for screening, diagnosis or staging of breast cancer. However, they can be useful in determining metastatic disease (Molina et al., 1999; Bast et al., 2001).

Prostate-specific antigen (PSA) is another controversial marker due to false positive and false negative results when used as a screening test, and it is not recommended for screening in the United Kingdom. If used as a screening test for men over 50 years old, or those at high risk due to a family history of prostate cancer, further investigation should be included (Lamerz et al., 1999; Semjonow et al., 1999; American Urological Association, 2000).

The Future Role of Tumour Markers in Disease Management

Since 1997, the National Cancer Institute in the United States has provided major funding for research on new diagnostic, prognostic and predictive cancer markers, as well as for translating research techniques which have been used on cell lines or animal models into clinical use, to assist oncologists in selecting correct treatment strategies.

Completion of the Human Genome Project has provided sequence data and advanced into the next stage of identifying the expressed products of these genes (Collins *et al.,* 1998).

The National Cancer Institute (NCI) has established the Cancer Genome Anatomy Project (CGAP), which is developing a catalogue of genes associated with cancer. This resource reads the molecular signatures/portraits of cancer from mRNA by extracting good quality DNA and mRNA from archived tumour formalin fixed paraffin embedded tissue (FFPE), a procedure previously thought impossible. This is used with microarray (gene) chips and real-time PCR and compared with normal tissue to find those tissues with increased or decreased expressions of specific mRNAs (Strausberg *et al.,* 1997, 2000). Over 4 500 000 gene sequence tags have been deposited in this public bioinformatics cDNA library database, together with their histological reports, TNM staging and clinical outcome data (Lal *et al.,* 1999; Strausberg, 2001).

Work has been undertaken to identify proteins associated with the expressed mRNA, using a proteomics approach. One of the main aims was to identify suitable early detection cancer markers and other markers for prognosis. The results of clinical studies, using existing tumour markers, provide information on which markers are the best to use (NCI, 2005).

Protein chips, surface-enhanced laser desorption/ionization (SLEDI) and mass spectrometry (MS) detection are being used to compare protein-fingerprint profiles of paired normal and tumour tissues. These techniques may, in the future, identify new tumour markers that can be used in early detection.

The next few years will see multiplexed antibody sandwich immunoassay as microarrays being introduced into clinical laboratories. These immunoassay chips will include miniaturized versions of existing tumour assays, allowing multiplex testing on small sample volumes with high throughput systems, contributing to an economical tumour profiling approach for patients with cancer.

Other approaches include the detection of circulating tumour cells in patients' blood and examination of circulating autoantibodies raised against the tumour markers themselves. In patients with cancer, these autoantibodies would be more prevalent than in cancer-free individuals. In the case of MUC-1, serial serum samples from patients with primary breast cancer showed significant correlation between tissue staining and circulating autoantibodies. The use of multiple biomarkers, due to the heterogeneous nature of cancers, can increase the sensitivity of tumour markers (Cheung *et al.,* 2002).

The use of anti-angiogenesis therapy for the treatment of cancer is becoming a favoured approach. Rather than eradicate the tumour, the therapy aims to send the tumour into dormancy. Such therapy will need to be sustained for long periods and patients will require monitoring for both inhibitor and pro-angiogenesis factors on a regular basis (Folkman, Browder and Palmblad, 2001; Kerbel and Folkman, 2002).

10 Monoclonal Antibodies

HELMOUT MODJTAHEDI

BACKGROUND

Cancer is the leading cause of death in developed countries (Parkin, 2001). Despite major advances in chemotherapy, treatment with cytotoxic drugs, in particular of metastatic solid tumours, does not induce complete remission in the great majority of patients (Tzioras et al., 2006). As cytotoxic drugs are not specific for tumour cells, there is often a wide range of toxicity associated with their use. The development of drug resistant phenotypes is a major cause of treatment failure. Therefore, identification of antigens which play important roles in tumour pathogenesis and targeting of such antigens with specific anticancer drugs is essential if we are to win the battle against cancer. Since the 1900s, one major goal of scientists has been the production of large amounts of a single type of antibody against a tumour antigen, which could be used as a 'magic bullet' in the treatment of cancer (Dillman, 1989; Ward, Hawkins and Smith, 1997; Gura, 2002; Harris, 2004).

In 1975, Köhler and Milstein developed a procedure called hybridoma technology for the production of monoclonal antibodies in mice. This technology, which allows the production of unlimited quantities of a specific type of antibody (monoclonal antibody or mAb) against any target antigen, has revolutionized many areas of biological and medical research. As a result of the specificity of a particular mAb for a particular antigen, mAbs have been generated against a wide range of antigens in the past 30 years. Monoclonal antibodies have become essential tools in the furthering of our understanding of the function of many genes and their protein products, in the discovery of novel tumour antigens, in the diagnosis of cancers and in tumour classification. In addition, as a result of recent advances in genetic engineering and of our better understanding of cancer biology, tumour antigens and tumour immunology, monoclonal antibodies are now being used for the treatment of cancer patients (Waldman, 2003; Sharkey and Goldberg, 2006).

Since 1992, 12 antibodies have been approved by the US Food and Drug Administration (FDA) for the detection and management of human cancers (Gura, 2002; Sharkey and Goldberg, 2006).

Of these, six unconjugated mAbs have been approved for the treatment of human cancers. Other mAbs have been conjugated to other therapeutic agents such as

The Biology of Cancer, Second Edition. Edited by J. Gabriel
© 2007 John Wiley & Sons, Ltd.

Table 10.1 Monoclonal antibodies that have been approved by the US Food and Drug Administration for cancer therapy

Antibody Name	Target Antigen	Antibody Format	Therapeutic Area	Year
Rituximab (Rituxan)	CD20	Chimeric (mouse-human IgG1)	Non-Hodgkin's lymphoma	1997
Trastuzumab (Herceptin)	HER-2	Humanized (IgG1)	Metastatic breast cancer;	1998
			Early breast cancer	2006
Gemtuzumab ozogamicin (Mylotarg)	CD33	Humanized (IgG1) (attached to toxin)	Acute myeloid leukaemia	2000
Alemtuzumab (Campath 1H)	CD52	Humanized (IgG1)	Chronic lymphocytic leukaemia	2001
Ibritumomab tiuxetan (Zevalin)	CD20	Mouse (attached to yttrium-90)	Non-Hodgkin's lymphoma	2002
Tosituzumab (Bexxar)	CD20	Mouse (attached to iodine-131)	Non-Hodgkin's lymphoma	2003
Bevacizumab (Avastin)	VEGF	Humanized (mouse-human IgG1)	Metastatic colorectal cancer	2004
Erbitux (Cetuximab)	EGFR	Chimeric (mouse-human IgG1)	Metastatic colorectal cancer;	2004
			Head and neck cancer	2006
Panitumumab (Vectibix)	EGFR	Human (IgG2)	Metastatic colorectal cancer	2006

radioisotopes and drugs in order to increase the specific delivery of such agents to tumour cells (Table 10.1). Currently, mAbs account for about 30% of all new biotechnology drugs in development, with more than 400 at different stages of clinical trial worldwide (Pavlou and Belsey, 2005).

In this chapter, the structure and function of mAbs (naked and conjugated) are discussed, together with the principles of their therapeutic application. Recent advances in mAb technology and our understanding of tumour antigens, which have led to the current use of mAbs in the management of human cancers, are also covered. There is particular focus on a number of mAbs, such as trastuzumab and rituximab, which are currently used in the treatment of metastatic breast cancer and haematological malignancies, and cetuximab, which has proven efficacy in the treatment of metastatic colorectal cancer and head and neck cancer.

WHAT ARE ANTIBODIES AND MONOCLONAL ANTIBODIES?

Antibodies are immunoglobulins (Igs) that are produced after the exposure of activated B-lymphocytes to a particular antigen (Figure 10.1). They are Y-shaped structures that are present on the surface of B-lymphocytes or circulate in the bloodstream after secretion by a differentiated form of B-lymphocytes called plasma cells. All antibodies have the same basic structure and consist of two identical heavy (H) chains and two identical light (L) chains which are held together by disulfide bonds (Figure 10.1(a)). Both heavy chains and light chains are further divided into variable (V) or constant (C) regions. The variable portion of both the heavy and

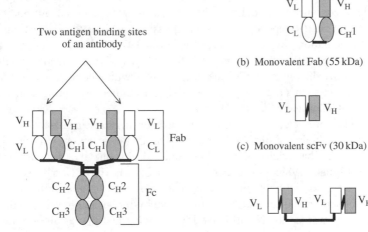

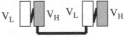

Figure 10.1 Structure of an intact antibody (immunoglobulin) and an antibody fragment developed by genetic engineering for tumour imaging and therapeutic applications. An intact antibody consists of two identical heavy chains and two identical light chains connected by disulfide (−S−S−) bonds (a). Both heavy (larger) chains and light (smaller) chains contain a constant portion (CH and CL, respectively) and a variable portion (VH and VL, respectively). The antigen-binding site of an antibody is located at the variable domain of the antibody (i.e. VH and VL) and the antibody's immunological effect is mediated by the constant (Fc) portion of the antibody. To increase tumour penetration, smaller fragments of antibodies, such as monovalent Fab, scFv or divalent (scFv)2, have been generated, which retain the antigen-binding specificity of the intact antibody. (a) Intact divalent IgG molecule (150 kDa); (b) monovalent Fab (55 kDa); (c) monovalent scFv (30 kDa); and (d) divalent (scFv)2 (60 kDa).

light chains (VH and VL) forms the two identical antigen-binding fragments (Fab) of the antibody. The constant portions of the heavy chains, called crystallizable fragments (Fc), are responsible for the activation of the complement system and for alerting the host immune system to attack the target antigen (Spiridon, Guinn and Vitetta, 2004).

One of the useful characteristics of antibodies is that they are extremely specific for a particular antigen. Before 1975, antibodies were generated by the repeated immunization of a group of animals with a particular antigen (e.g. viruses, bacteria, tumour cells). Sera were collected from the animals and used for the treatment of patients who had the same infection. Unfortunately, the administration of the crude preparation of sera, which also contained other animal proteins, produced strong allergic reactions in many patients. In addition, when a recipient animal (e.g. a sheep, a rabbit or a mouse) is immunized with an antigen, the serum from such an animal contains a mixture of different antibodies. These antibodies, which are produced by different populations of B-lymphocytes, are called polyclonal antibodies. The serum may therefore contain very low levels of therapeutic antibodies (Ward, Hawkins and Smith, 1997). Furthermore, as a result of the short survival of B-lymphocytes from immunized animals in culture, the large-scale production of antibodies from a single clone of B-lymphocytes was not possible – until the innovation of the hybridoma technology by Köhler and Milstein in 1975. Using this technology, the antibody-producing B-lymphocytes from the spleens of immunized animals were immortalized by the fusion of their cell membranes with a continuous proliferation of myeloma cells, in order to produce a single antibody-secreting cell called a hybridoma (Köhler and Milstein, 1975).

Using hybridoma technology, mAbs have been prepared against a wide range of antigens, including growth factors, growth factor receptors, tumour-specific antigens, viruses, bacterial products, hormones, drugs, enzymes and differentiated antigens (Dillman, 1989; Ward, Hawkins and Smith, 1997; Harris, 2004). Such antibodies are used routinely in the identification of such antigens in human tumour biopsies and sera, and in investigating their role in tumour progression. Köhler and Milstein were awarded the Nobel Prize for Medicine in 1984, as a consequence of the great impact of hybridoma technology on medical sciences.

ENGINEERED ANTIBODIES

These include chimeric antibodies, humanized antibodies, human antibodies and antibody fragments. The first panel of monoclonal antibodies was developed against human tumour antigens in mice (Köhler and Milstein, 1975). Although mouse antibodies are very useful as diagnostic agents and in the unravelling of the biological and clinical significance of human tumour antigens, their therapeutic application in patients may be limited because of their immunogenicity (Dillman, 1989; Coghlan, 1991). When repeated doses of antibodies from a non-human source (e.g. mouse antibodies) are given to patients, such antibodies may be recognized as 'foreign' by the patients' immune systems and lead to the generation of a human anti-mouse antibody (HAMA) response (Ward, Hawkins and Smith, 1997). This in turn may lead to the elimination of the administered antibody from the patient's bloodstream before any therapeutic effects can be produced (Dillman, 1989; Ward, Hawkins and Smith, 1997).

CHIMERIC AND HUMANIZED ANTIBODIES

Following advances in genetic engineering in the 1980s and 1990s, the immunogenicity of mouse antibodies has been reduced by several methods (Hudson and Souriau, 1993). The chimeric format of mouse antibodies has been developed by transferring the antigen-binding domain (VH and VL) of mouse antibodies into a human IgG framework (Figure 10.2). Chimeric antibodies, which are a 30:70 mixture of mouse and human sequences, are expected to be less immunogenic than mouse antibodies (see Rituximab). Humanized versions of mouse antibodies have also been developed by transferring three stretches of amino acids in the variable

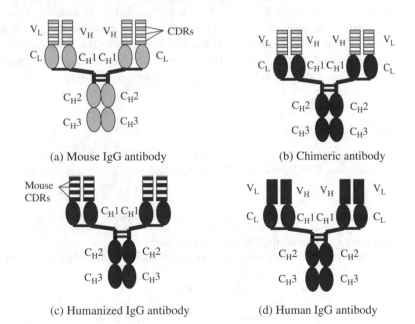

(a) Mouse IgG antibody   (b) Chimeric antibody

(c) Humanized IgG antibody   (d) Human IgG antibody

Figure 10.2 Structure of (a) mouse (first generation, 1970s), (b) chimeric (second generation, 1980s) and (c, d) humanized (third generation, 1990s) monoclonal antibodies developed for therapeutic applications. The chimeric monoclonal antibodies contain 66% human sequence and 34% mouse (VH and VL) sequence and are generated by the fusion of DNA from the mouse variable region to DNA from a constant region of human IgG antibody. In contrast, humanized antibodies contain more than 90% of human sequences and are formed by fusion of DNA from three stretches of amino acids in the mouse variable domain into a human IgG framework.

region of mouse antibodies (CDRs), which are responsible for the binding to the antigen, into the human IgG framework (Figure 10.2). The resultant humanized antibodies contain more human sequences (90%) and should be less immunogenic than mouse and chimeric antibodies in cancer patients (see 'Trastuzumab'). Most clinical trials currently under way use the chimeric or humanized form of mouse antibodies (Hudson and Souriau, 1993; Pavlou and Belsey, 2005) (Table 10.2).

HUMAN MONOCLONAL ANTIBODIES

Since the early 1990s, and as a result of advances in molecular biology, it has become possible to develop fully human mAbs against human tumour antigens (Winter and Milstein, 1991; Marks and Marks, 1996; Glover, 1999; Davies, Gallo and Corvalan, 1999; Pavlou and Belsey, 2005). The two techniques for the development of human antibodies against human antigens are the phage display technology and the use of transgenic mice – XenoMouse animals. In the latter case, in these animals, the mouse antibody gene has been replaced by a human antibody gene. The immunization of transgenic mice with human tumour antigens has led to the development of human antibodies in such animals. Clinical trials with a number of fully human mAbs are currently under way worldwide (Gibson, Ranganathan and Grothey, 2006). The results should indicate whether chronic (i.e. repeated) treatment of cancer patients with human mAbs is more effective and less immunogenic than treatment with chimeric antibodies or humanized mAbs directed against the same tumour antigen.

ANTIBODY FRAGMENTS

Preclinical and clinical studies with radiolabelled antibodies have indicated that intact antibodies such as whole IgG (160 kDa) are too large for rapid penetration

Table 10.2   Mechanisms by which monoclonal antibodies produce therapeutic effects

---

(a) Unconjugated (i.e. unmodified) monoclonal antibodies
   – by blocking the binding of growth factors to their receptors, which is essential for
     tumour proliferation
   – by inducing programmed cell death (i.e. apoptosis)
   – by binding to effector cells (e.g. natural killer or NK cells) and inducing
     antibody-dependent cellular cytotoxicity (ADCC) at the tumour sites
   – by activating complement and inducing complement-dependent cytotoxicity (CDC)
**(b) Conjugated monoclonal antibodies: by attachment to the following agents, a lethal
   dose of such molecules can be delivered to tumour cells:**
   – toxins (e.g. diphtheria toxin, pseudomonas exotoxin)
   – radioisotope (e.g. iodine-131, yttrium-90)
**(c) Bispecific mAbs: enhance tumour destruction by host immune effector function
   (e.g. MDX-210)**

---

of solid tumours and have slow blood clearance (Green, Murray and Hortobagi, 2000; Gura, 2002). With advances in genetic engineering, smaller fragments of the antibodies, such as Fab (55 kDa) and scFv (30 kDa), have been developed to retain a single antigen-binding fragment (i.e. monovalent) of the intact divalent antibody (see Figure 10.1(b)–(d)). Smaller fragments of such antibodies can be attached to radioisotopes for *in vivo* imaging or therapy of tumours, because they can penetrate tissue more effectively and clear faster from a patient's peripheral circulation (Hudson and Souriau, 1993).

THE MECHANISM OF ACTION OF MONOCLONAL ANTIBODIES

As each antibody is highly specific for a particular antigen, they have found widespread use in diagnostic kits, basic research and, more recently, cancer management (see below). In addition, after the recent success in mapping the human genome, mAb technology has become an essential tool in the discovery of novel human tumour antigens that are overexpressed in human malignancies, and in the identification of antigens that are differentially expressed between the primary and metastatic tumours (Holt *et al.*, 2000).

Depending on the subclass (Fc portion) of antibodies, and the antigens recognized by such antibodies, mAbs can produce their anti-tumour activities by several mechanisms (see Table 10.2). Monoclonal antibodies can inhibit the growth of tumours by blocking the binding of growth factors, which are essential for tumour cell proliferation, to such receptors (e.g. anti-EGFR antibody cetuximab; Mendelsohn, 2001). Monoclonal antibodies can also induce anti-tumour activity *in vivo* by directing ADCC and mediating CDC (Ward, Hawkins and Smith, 1997) (see Chapter 6). Of human IgGs, IgG1 antibodies are ideal for inducing ADCC at tumour sites, by binding to human mononuclear NK cells and macrophages. When a human IgG1 antibody binds to a target antigen on the tumour cell surface, via their Fab domain, the Fc portion of such antibodies can also bind to Fc receptors on circulating NK cells and macrophages. The binding of such immune cells to antibodies at the tumour sites can mediate ADCC in such target cells. The results of preclinical studies with a panel of mAbs have shown that the anti-tumour activity of mAbs improves substantially *in vivo*, when such antibodies could also trigger ADCC by bringing cytotoxic T-lymphocytes, NK cells and other immune effector cells to the tumour sites (Carter *et al.*, 1992; Ward *et al*, 1997).

As explained above, each antibody molecule has two identical antigen-binding domains. To enhance the effector function of an antibody, bispecific mAbs have been generated, which are directed against two different target antigens, with one arm binding to the antigen on host immune cells (e.g. CD3 antigen on T-cells) (Booy *et al.*, 2006). A number of phase 2/3 clinical trials with different bispecific mAbs are currently under way in several clinics worldwide. The results of such trials should unravel the full potential of this new approach in cancer therapy (Cao and Lam, 2003; Booy *et al.,* 2006).

In other cases, mAbs have been attached to cytotoxic drugs, radioisotopes or enzymes in order to deliver the lethal doses of such molecules to tumour cells or for use in tumour imaging (Pagliargo *et al.,* 1998; Dillman, 2002; Fracasso *et al.,* 2002; Pastan *et al.,* 2006). Ideally in such cases, the antigen should be overexpressed on malignant tumours, with no, or a very low level of, expression in normal tissues.

The characteristics of ideal antigens as targets for mAb-based therapy are given below:

- overexpression of target antigens on tumour cell surfaces;
- no or limited level of expression of antigens on normal cell surfaces;
- homogeneous expression of antigens on tumour cells; and
- no shedding of tumour antigens in patients' sera, which can trap the administered therapeutic antibody progression.

MONOCLONAL ANTIBODIES THAT ARE CURRENTLY USED IN CANCER THERAPY

There are currently nine mAbs commercially available that have been approved for the treatment of haematological cancers and breast, colorectal and head and neck cancers (see Table 10.1). The characteristic features of these antibodies, together with the antigens recognized by them, are discussed below.

RITUXIMAB

Rituximab was the first monoclonal antibody to be approved by the US FDA for the treatment of cancer, in 1997. Rituximab is a chimeric mAb (34% mouse protein and 66% human protein) and is directed against B-lymphocyte-restricted differentiation antigen CD20. It has been developed by transferring the entire Fab domain of mouse anti-CD20 antibody to the human IgG1 framework (Hainsworth, 2000). CD-20 antigen is expressed on the surface of more than 90% of B-cell non-Hodgkin's lymphomas (NHLs), on pre-B-lymphocytes and on mature lymphocytes, but not on stem cells, plasma cells or other normal tissues. B-cell lymphoma accounts for 95% of all lymphomas. Rituximab is jointly marketed by two American companies (IDEC Pharmaceutical and Genentech, California) for short-course outpatient treatment of relapsed or refractory CD20-positive, low-grade or follicular B-cell NHL. Rituximab is a less toxic alternative to chemotherapy and can induce anticancer activity by binding to CD20-positive cells, inducing apoptosis, recruiting immune effector functions (i.e. mediating ADCC) and activating complement (Scott, 1998; Hainsworth, 2000). As a single agent, rituximab has been shown to produce a response rate of 50% in patients with relapsed low-grade and follicular NHL. When added to standard chemotherapy in patients with diffuse, large B-cell NHL, it has been shown to prolong survival (Dearden, 2002). Treatment-related toxicity, which occurs most often with the first infusion of the antibody, is generally mild. Infusion-related reactions included rigors, nausea, urticaria, fatigue and headache (Dillman, 2002). One advantage of rituximab therapy is that, as it induces minimal adverse effects, it can be given to patients as short-course, outpatient therapy (375 mg/m^2 weekly for 4−8 weeks).

The mAbs epratuzumab and apolizumab, which are directed against two different antigens, CD22 and HLD-DR respectively, are also under clinical investigation for use in NHL (Leonard and Link, 2002). Simultaneous targeting of CD20, CD22 and HLA-DR antigens by antibodies in patients with NHL may produce a better therapeutic benefit, compared with treatment by one antibody. Further clinical trials in patients with NHL, with a combination of rituximab, epratuzumab and apolizumab, should unravel the full potential of such strategies (Sharkey and Goldenberg, 2006).

TRASTUZUMAB (HERCEPTIN)

Trastuzumab was the first therapeutic monoclonal antibody that was approved by the US FDA for the treatment of solid tumours, in 1998 (Freebairn, Last and Illidge, 2001; Bell, 2002). Unlike rituximab, trastuzumab is a humanized antibody. It is directed against the external domain of the human epidermal growth factor receptor 2 (HER-2). It has been approved for the treatment of patients with metastatic breast cancer whose tumours overexpress HER-2 receptors. HER-2 is a non-mutated, tumour-associated, cell-surface antigen and a member of the type I growth factor receptor family (Rubin and Yarden, 2001). Overexpression of HER-2 has been shown in 20−30% of patients with breast cancer and in a number of other epithelial tumours (Walker, 2000). High levels of expression of HER-2 have often been associated with more aggressive disease, poor response to the conventional form of therapy, increased risk of metastasis and poor survival in patients with breast cancer (Cook et al., 2001). As HER-2 overexpression plays an important role in the clinical behaviour of human tumours and is responsible for a poor response to conventional forms of therapy, it forms an ideal target for mAb-based therapy (Green, Murray and Hortobagi, 2000; Rubin and Yarden, 2001).

In the past 18 years, a panel of mouse and rat mAbs has been generated against the external domain of HER-2 for both diagnostic and therapeutic applications in oncology (Sliwkowski et al., 1999; Baselga and Albanell, 2001). HER-2 blockade by mAbs has been shown to inhibit the proliferation of the HER-2-overexpressing tumours, both in vitro and in animal models (Baselga and Albanell, 2001). The mouse anti-HER-2 mAb 4D5, which showed potent anti-tumour activity and specificity in preclinical studies, was selected for humanization by the American biotech company Genentech (Carter et al., 1992). The humanized form of mouse anti-HER-2 mAb 4D5 (i.e. trastuzumab) was generated by transferring the CDR from mAb 4D5 into a human IgG1 framework (Carter et al., 1992). Preclinical studies with trastuzumab have shown that it can induce anti-tumour activity against HER-2-overexpressing tumours by several mechanisms, including downregulation of HER-2 from the cell surface and its subsequent mitogenic signal, cell-cycle arrest, induction of apoptosis, inhibition of angiogenesis, activation of complement and mediation of ADCC at tumour sites – by binding to effector cells such as NK cells (Sliwkowski *et al.*, 1999; Harries and Smith, 2002). In addition, trastuzumab has been shown to increase the anti-tumour activity of cytotoxic drugs against HER-2-overexpressing human breast tumour cell lines in preclinical settings (Baselga *et al.*, 1998; Sliwkowski *et al.*, 1999; Baselga and Albanell, 2001). Clinical trials with trastuzumab, both as a single agent and in combination with cytotoxic drugs such as paclitaxel, have shown that it improves survival in breast cancer patients (Harries and Smith, 2002). The benefit was most evident in patients whose tumours expressed the highest level of HER-2 (3+). The results of clinical studies have also indicated that, although trastuzumab is well tolerated in the great majority of patients, cardiac toxicity is seen in a minority (about 2%) of those treated with trastuzumab alone, and in 26–28% of those who received trastuzumab in combination with an anthracycline regimen. In addition, recent studies have indicated that some cancer patients whose tumours are HER-2 positive may shed some HER-2 antigen into their sera (Hait, 2001). Such shed antigens may trap some of the administered trastuzumab, reducing the effective dose reaching the tumour sites. In such cases, the dose of trastuzumab administered to patients should be increased to compensate for the antibodies trapped by shed antigens.

More recently, in some studies Herceptin was also found to improve disease-free survival among women with HER-2 positive breast cancer in the adjuvant setting (i.e. after excision of early-breast cancer) (Norum, 2006). On 16 November 2006, the FDA expanded the use of trastuzumab, in combination with other drugs, for the treatment of early-stage HER-2-positive breast cancer after surgery (www.fda.gov/).

ALEMTUZUMAB

Alemtuzumab is a humanized mAb that is directed against the CD52 antigen (Waldman, 2002). The CD52 antigen is present on the surface of normal T-lymphocytes, B-lymphocytes and a high proportion of lymphoid cancers, but absent on haematopoietic stem cells. The original rat monoclonal antibody against CD52 was generated in Cambridge, in the United Kingdom, in 1980, and the humanized version of this antibody was approved by the FDA for the treatment of B-cell chronic lymphocytic leukaemia (CLL) in patients who have failed fludarabine therapy (Waldman, 2002). This antibody is able to 'kill' CD52-positive target cells by activating complement and by mediating ADCC (Dearden, 2002; Foran, 2002; Waldman, 2002; Ferrajoli, Faderi and Keating, 2006). However, this antibody induces immunosuppression, as a result of depletion of normal B- and T-lymphocytes, causing an increased risk of opportunistic infections (Pangalis *et al.*, 2001; Rai *et al.*, 2002).

CETUXIMAB AND PANITUMUMAB

Cetuximab is a chimeric, and panitumumab a fully human monoclonal antibody directed against the external domain of human epidermal growth factor receptor

(EGFR), which were approved by the FDA for the treatment of colorectal cancer (www.fda.gov/). The EGFR transmits the mitogenic action of the EGF family of growth factors, such as EGF, transforming growth factor TGFα, HB-EGF (heparin-binding epidermal growth factor), BTC (betacellulin) and epiregulin (Modjtahedi and Dean, 1994; Mendelsohn, 2001). From histological examination of human tumour biopsies, it has become evident that overexpression of EGFR, accompanied by co-production of one or more of its ligands, is a common feature of human tumours of epithelial origin (Modjtahedi and Dean, 1994). Overexpression of EGFR has been detected in cancer of the bladder, breast, lung, brain, stomach, prostate, ovary, pancreas and head and neck. It has been associated with a poor prognosis, as well as resistance to chemotherapy and/or radiotherapy, in many patients with these cancers (Modjtahedi and Dean, 1994; Nicholson, Gee and Harper, 2001). Consequently, several laboratories have generated a panel of mAbs against the external domain of EGFR, which blocks the binding of the ligands to EGFR and inhibits the growth *in vitro* and *in vivo* of a wide range of human tumours that overexpress EGFR (Modjtahedi *et al.*, 1996; Mendelsohn, 2001; Yang *et al.*, 2001; Needle, 2002). The anti-tumour activities of anti-EGFR antibodies have been shown to be mediated via several mechanisms, including down-regulation of the EGFR from the tumour cell surface, induction of G1 arrest, promotion of apoptosis, inhibition of angiogenesis and immune activation, such as ADCC and CDC. On the basis of these findings, the anti-EGFR mAb cetuximab was approved by the US FDA for the treatment of metastatic colorectal cancer in combination with chemotherapy (February 2004) and in combination with radiotherapy for the treatment of head and neck cancer (March 2006). The improved response rate and survival benefit does, however, come at a price. An estimated cost of treatment with cetuximab, with a loading dose of 450 mg/m^2 in the first week and followed by weekly dose of 250 mg/m^2 per patient for an eight week duration, is around \$20 300 (Schrag, 2004). A further challenge in the routine use of anti-EGFR antibodies in the treatment of cancer patients is the identification of more specific tumour markers that can be used not only in the selection of a more specific subpopultaion of EGFR-positive patients who benefit from therapy with anti-EGFR antibodies, but also in discovering those factors that are responsible for the poor response or the development of resistance to therapy with anti-EGFR antibodies.

In September 2006, the FDA approved the fully human anti-EGFR antibody panitumumab for the treatment of patients with EGFR expressing non-curable metastatic colorectal carcinoma (Gibson, Ranganathan and Grothey, 2006). As panitumumab is a fully human anti-EGFR monoclonal antibody, patients receiving this antibody will run a reduced risk of developing an allergic reaction, compared to those receiving the chimeric anti-EGFR antibody cetuximab.

BEVACIZUMAB

Angiogenesis, the formation of new blood vessels, has been shown to be essential for the local growth of tumour cells (Folkman, 1992). High levels of angiogenesis have been associated with a poor prognosis in many patients with epithelial tumours.

Bevacizumab is a humanized monoclonal antibody, and was the first angiogenesis inhibitor to be approved by the FDA as the first line treatment for patients with metastatic colorectal cancer, in combination with standard chemotherapy (Culy, 2005). In combination with cytotoxic agents, bevacizumab increased overall survival by 5 months and median progression-free survival by 4 months, compared to cytotoxic drugs alone. Bevacizumab inhibits tumour growth by blocking the function of vascular endothelial growth factor (VEGF), a potent mitogen, and survival factor for endothelial cells. Recent studies suggest that bevacizumab may also have potential in treatment of other cancers, such as renal cell cancer and ovarian, lung and breast cancers (Ellis, 2005). The two most common side effects reported with this drug are hypertension and blood clots. There were also rare reports of bowel perforation.

CONJUGATED MONOCLONAL ANTIBODIES IN CANCER THERAPY

As explained above, in some cases mAbs have been attached to modified toxins or radioisotopes in order to deliver lethal doses of such molecules to tumour cells. Ideal antigens for such therapeutic strategies are tumour-specific antigens. Three conjugated mAbs that have been approved for the treatment of human cancers are described here.

IMMUNOTOXIN: GEMTUZUMAB OZOGAMICIN (MYLOTARG)

Gemtuzumab ozogamicin is the first toxin-linked antibody to be approved for the treatment of human cancer. It is a humanized anti-CD33 mAb which is attached to the cytotoxic anti-tumour antibiotic calicheamicin (Berger *et al.,* 2002). It has been approved by the US FDA as a single agent for the treatment of patients with CD33-positive acute myeloid leukaemia (AML) in the first relapse who are over the age of 60 and not suitable for therapy with conventional cytotoxic drugs (Berger *et al.,* 2002; Dearden, 2002). AML is the most common type of acute leukaemia in adults and is characterized by accumulation and proliferation of myeloblasts in the bone marrow.

The CD33 antigen is not expressed on stem cells or non-haematopoietic normal cells, but has been shown to be expressed on myeloblasts in 80–90% of patients with AML. The binding of this immunotoxin to CD33 antigen on AML cells results in the internalization of the immunotoxin and dissociation of calicheamicin; its transport into the nucleus and the following degradation of the DNA lead ultimately to cell death. Clinical studies with Mylotarg, as a single agent in patients with CD33-positive AML, produced a complete response rate of 15–20% (Berger *et al.,* 2002). A potential complication of therapy associated with Mylotarg is the increased risk of veno-occlusive disease, even without bone marrow transplantation (Abutalib and Tallman, 2006).

RADIOLABELLED mAbs AS RADIOIMMUNOCONJUGATE AGENTS: IBRITUMOMAB TIUXETAN (ZEVALIN) AND TOSITUZUMAB (BEXXAR)

The goal of radioimmunotherapy (RIT) is to deliver cytotoxic radiation from therapeutic radioisotopes to tumours using mAbs (similar to a guided missile) that bind to those cells expressing the target antigen (Hainsworth, 2000; Cheson, 2001). The success of RIT depends on several factors, including the choice of the target antigens, antibody molecules (guided missiles) and therapeutic radioisotopes (Juweid, 2002). Ideally the target antigen should be tumour specific and expressed only on tumour cells, with no level of expression on normal cells. In practice, most of the target antigens recognized by antibodies are tumour-associated antigens that are also present in lower numbers on the surface of normal cells. To minimize exposure of such normal cells to the radioisotope, a relatively high dose of unlabelled antibody is given to patients, either before or during the administration of the various radiolabelled antibodies. The two most common isotopes that are used in RIT are iodine-131 (131I) and yttrium-90 (90Y) (Dillman, 2002; Juweid, 2002). The advantage of radioimmunotherapy over unconjugated antibodies in cancer therapy is that the former has a longer path, which allows further, deeper penetration and killing of tumour cells (both antigen positive and negative), without direct binding of the antibodies to such tumours (Sharkey and Goldberg, 2006).

Ibritumomab tiuxetan was the first RIT agent to be approved for the treatment of cancer, in February 2002 (Dillman, 2002). It is a 90Y-labelled anti-CD20 antibody (IDEC Pharmaceuticals, US) which has been shown to produce a 74% response rate in Rituxan-refractory NHL patients. To determine the relative efficacy of ibritumomab tiuxetan (90Y-labelled anti-CD20 antibody), compared to unconjugated anti-CD20 antibody rituximab, in the treatment of patients with NHL, 143 NHL patients were randomized into two groups, in a phase 3 clinical trial. The overall response rate in patients treated with ibritumomab tiuxetan was 80%, compared with 56% in those treated with rituximab. As explained above, the advantage of RIT over unconjugated mAb is that the former penetrates deeper into the tumour mass; it can also kill antigen-negative tumours in a crossfire effect. Therefore, patients who are not responsive to, or relapse after chemotherapy or treatment with unconjugated antibodies, may be suitable candidates for RIT approaches (Dillman, 2002; Foran, 2002; Juweid, 2002).

Tosituzumab (Bexxar) was the second anti-CD20 monoclonal antibody conjugated to iodine-131 to be approved by the FDA, in 2003, for the treatment of refractory NHL (DeNardo, Sysko and DeNardo, 2006). To facilitate rapid clearance and so reduce the duration of total body irradiation, both radiolabelled antibodies (Bexxar and Zevalin) are of mouse origin. They both prolong survival rate in Rituxan-refractory NHL patients (Sharkey and Goldenberg, 2006).

The full details of antibody-based products that have been approved by the FDA for clinical use in cancer and other pathological conditions can be found by visiting the FDA's web site: www.fda.gov/.

CONCLUSION

Since the discovery of hybridoma technology, mAbs have been generated against a wide range of human tumour antigens and have been used to unravel the importance of such antigens in the biology of cancer. These antibodies have also been used as diagnostic agents and, more recently, in cancer treatment. Unfortunately, the first generation of mAbs, which were generated in mice, were immunogenic in cancer patients. This prevented their repeated administration, limiting their efficacy. Following advances in genetic engineering, it has become possible to develop the recombinant form of mice monoclonal antibodies (i.e. chimeric or humanized). Six such unconjugated antibodies are currently being used in the management of cancer patients, because they prolong survival. More importantly, patients treated with mAbs do not develop high-grade side effects, which are often associated with the use of conventional chemotherapy. In some cases, the anti-tumour activity of mAbs has been enhanced by conjugating to toxins and radioisotopes in order to deliver lethal doses of such molecules to tumour cells. Although antibodies such as rituximab, trastuzumab and cetuximab are very useful in the treatment of cancer patients, the duration of response in some patients may be short (less than a year) (Schrag, 2004). In addition, the chronic use of certain antibodies for treatment of cancer patients is currently very expensive. Therefore, with the identification of other cell-surface antigens of biological and clinical significance, and by simultaneous targeting of such antigens with antibodies and other therapeutic strategies, it should be possible to prolong survival in most cancer patients and to reduce cost by reducing the need for frequent administration of antibody-based drugs. The results of ongoing clinical trials of hundreds of mAbs, which are directed against a wide range of human antigens, will illustrate the full potential of monoclonal antibody-based products as 'magic bullets' in the treatment of human cancer.

Part III From Research to Treatment

11 What is Translational Oncology Research?

ELAINE LENNAN

'Is it something to do with genetics?' 'Is it about converting something into some-thing else?' 'Haven't got a clue.' In fact all three are correct. Translational oncology research is a fairly new term. The *Concise Oxford English Dictionary* (Allen, 1990) describes translation as: 'the process of moving something from one place to another.' Many have similarly described translational oncology as 'bench to treatment couch'.

When thinking of cancer research, be it prevention, diagnosis or treatment, one tends to think of two areas: the laboratory-based researchers, that is scientists in white coats who inject test tubes or culture Petri dishes, and clinical trials where patients are directly involved in the testing of a substance or treatment. Translational oncology research aims to bring the two dimensions together and make the laboratory work relevant to clinical practice (www.smd.qmul.ac.uk).

WHAT EXACTLY IS TRANSLATIONAL ONCOLOGY RESEARCH?

Researchers in basic biomedical science strive to unravel the workings of a phys-iological process. They want to understand how things do or do not work. This is important and groundbreaking work, but many patients and health professionals could argue 'so what, if it doesn't improve clinical outcomes?' The information learnt will no doubt contribute to the enormous knowledge and evidence base and help in the understanding of individuals, but will it really impact on better cancer treatments?

Translational research attempts to bridge the gap between test tube and patient, to ensure that new scientific findings are translated into new developments, either diagnostically or therapeutically (www.smu.qmul.ac.uk).

The fundamental purpose of the research is improved clinical practice. Trans-lational research takes something from the scientific arena to a patient and brings

The Biology of Cancer, Second Edition. Edited by J. Gabriel
© 2007 John Wiley & Sons, Ltd.

back questions from the patient to the scientists. This is not as easy as it sounds. Scientists do not always regularly read medical journals and medics do not generally read scienctific journals. Blagosklomy (2002) agrees with this statement and urges that data published in scientific journals be translated into detailed treatment protocols which can be directly used by a doctor and tested in a clinical trial. His thoughts are not unique. Birmingham (2002) quotes Professor Nadler who states: 'I can't train the next generation because there is now an enormous amount of science and no one to bring it to patients.'

WHAT TRANSLATIONAL ONCOLOGY RESEARCH IS NOT

Those involved in the following are *not* examples of translational oncology researchers:

- cloning genes from a human cell line or tissue;
- studying human specimen profiles on chips;
- developing new classes of drugs;
- company-based phase 1 trials.

Those who *are* translational oncology researchers are, through their own work, attempting to (Birmingham, 2002):

- improve diagnosis for patients;
- improve the prognosis for patients;
- improve cancer prevention;
- conceive or execute new treatments.

Looking at the lists above, there is potential benefit in bringing the knowledge of the researchers in the first list together with that of the researchers in the second list.

HOW WILL BRINGING THE SCIENCES TOGETHER BE ACHIEVED?

Searching the Internet and libraries for examples of translational oncology research reveals not only individual examples of 'bench to treatment couch' research, but entire programmes of research, including a coordinated approach to the subject in the United Kingdom (DoH, 2006).

The National Translational Cancer Research Network (NTRAC) has been established to speed up the processes by which laboratory-based research becomes a therapeutic treatment that will benefit cancer patients. The NTRAC currently incorporates fourteen centres of scientific and clinical research, each being selected by the Department of Health and cancer stakeholders (Table 11.1). Funded by the Department of Health, translational oncology research is now high on political

Table 11.1 NTRAC centres of scientific research

NTRAC Centre	Network Speciality
Belfast	Immunology; molecular pathology
Birmingham	Immunotherapy; gene therapy
Cambridge Addenbrookes	Molecular pathology; bioinformatics
Cardiff Swansea	Pathology; haematology
Edinburgh	Public health; population informatics; chemoprevention
Glasgow Dundee	Gene therapy; molecular pharmacology; pharmacogenetics
Imperial College London	Functional imaging; gene therapy
Leeds Bradford	Molecular and cellular pathology
Manchester	Functional imaging
Newcastle	Small molecules
Oxford	Tumour angiogenesis
Royal Marsden Institute of Cancer Research	Molecular pathology; imaging
Southampton	Immunotherapy
University College London (UCL)	Immunotherapy; functional imaging; bioinformatics

agendas. Recent changes have continued this funding but now in collaboration and partnership with Cancer Research UK. The overall aims remain the same, being to increase (www.ntrac.org.uk:)

- the number of new treatments and diagnostic tests;
- the number of early clinical trials; and
- the number of patients across the country taking part in these trials.

Alongside this coordinated approach, many other centres exist in isolation that do equally valuable work. Their fundamental aim is to develop laboratory work into new therapies and, in so doing, improve outcomes for patients.

Before looking at specific examples of translational oncology research, it is worth while looking at the breadth of translational work. The following is taken from NTRAC (2006).

Within the remit of translational research, areas of work can include the following:

- Small molecules: research has provided considerable insight into the molecules and pathways involved in transforming a normal cell into a cancer cell (see Chapter 4). These *changes* are being examined by scientists in striving to develop drugs that will inhibit or regulate their abnormal activity. Cancer Research UK is leading the development of novel anticancer agent treatments emerging from cancer research.

- Gene therapy and cancer vaccines: viruses can be genetically modified to carry a tumour-specific antigen. These are currently being developed for a range of cancers. This work will test the hypothesis underpinning vaccine development and included in it are mechanistic biological endpoints such as virus distribution immunological evidence or induction of T-cell response (see Chapter 8).
- Novel diagnostics: new and improved technologies developed from the genome knowledge are helping in the search for novel diagnostic, prognostic and predictive factors. These techniques will help the clinician to sub-define disease and tailor therapy to the individual patient, that is select anticancer therapies on an individual basis rather than a population basis. Projects of this type require close collaboration between those scientists who developed the technology and the clinicians who manage specific cancers within the multidisciplinary team (see Chapter 9).
- Hypothesis testing in clinical communities: this could involve assembling national DNA or cancer tissue banks. This will enable the clinical community to search for genes, proteins or other molecules that contribute to the clinical behaviour of different cancers.

These examples are cited as being dynamic processes that depend on the fusion of expertise. The bench researcher fully integrates with the front-line clinician and vice versa. To bring the start of this chapter alive and demonstrate translational oncology in practice, it is useful to work through a couple of areas of research.

ANGIOGENESIS

Angiogenesis is one example of laboratory research translated into clinical practice. It is the growth of a new blood supply from pre-existing vasculature. The existing capillaries sprout new branches to serve and nurture the tumour. This is triggered by a protein known as tumour angiogenesis factor, and involves numerous biological activities (see Chapter 4) (Tortora and Grabowski, 2003). Preclinical studies have demonstrated the major role of angiogenesis in tumour growth and formation of metastases, which has led to the thinking that suppression of the blood supply suppresses the tumour (Pinedo and Salmon, 2000). Most cancer treatments have been targeted at killing the cell. Although treatments have been modified and refined over the past 50 years, the aim of treatment remains targeted at the same tumour cell. An understanding of angiogenesis and the notion that the tumour is angiogenesis or blood-supply dependent have led to the second target in cancer treatment − the newly formed capillaries.

As mentioned above, the current thinking is that cancer treatment targets the cancer cell to cause cell death. Folkman, Browder and Palmblad (2001) suggest that the cancer genome is clever in its make-up, continually mutating or changing at both primary (main) and distant (secondary or metastases) sites. This creates challenges for the clinical staff because eventually these changes will create a resistance to the drugs targeted at the cancer. In stark contrast, the cells that line the new capillaries at the tumour site are stable, with a virtually non-existent mutation or change rate. These cells, known as microvasculature endothelial cells, are needed for further tumour growth, which makes them a very powerful player in any malignant process. These endothelial cells not only supply oxygen and nutrients to the tumour; it is now known that they also provide a gateway for anti apoptotic factors, or anti-switch-off factors, and so protect the tumour by allowing its cells to go into mass production. Simply, what the above is saying is that we know that a tumour continually changes its make-up and that it is dependent on a blood supply. The ever-changing nature of the tumour cells may result in drug resistance. The blood supply remains constant, supplying nutrients so that the tumour thrives. Killing the blood supply will kill the tumour, whether or not mutated and drug resistant. This is the basis of this translational research (Figure 11.1). Preclinical and clinical work is ongoing. Centres use anti-angiogenesis agents alone and/or in combination with chemotherapy. The aim is to inhibit tumour growth, reduce metastases, prolong survival and improve quality of life (Pinedo and Salmon, 2000).

Is it possible to have concurrent use of cytotoxic chemotherapy and anti-angiogenic agents? If the blood supply is suppressed, how do the cytotoxic drugs reach the tumour? This is a valid concern, but one that has not yet been elucidated. Animal studies of lung cancer by Leicher, cited by Pinedo and Salmon (2000), demonstrated a synergistic effect. Combination therapy reduced not only the number of metastases but also the size of the metastases, providing evidence that anti-angiogenic therapies can improve treatment.

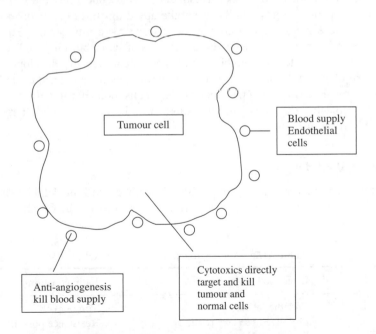

Figure 11.1 Targets for cell death.

How is Knowledge about Angiogenesis Changing Practice?

The cells that line the newly formed capillaries (microvasculature endothelial cells) supply the nutrients that encourage the tumour to thrive. Angiogenesis inhibitors are a new class of drug that work specifically to inhibit proliferating and migrating endothelial cells. Many of these drugs have now reached phase 3 trials. These drugs work in two ways and are summarized in Table 11.2. Currently there is no test or assay to determine the best approach/dose in an individual patient. The challenge for scientific researchers is to develop a simple test to measure the effects of angiogenesis inhibitors, which will aid clinicians in refining treatments to individual needs. It is hoped that, from this example, the role that scientists play in the quest to improve the outcome for the patient can be demonstrated; true 'bench to treatment couch' oncology research (Table 11.2).

IMATINIB MESYLATE

Another example of translational oncology research is one of the great successes of recent years, and that is the story of imatinib mesylate (Glivec). This has dramatically changed the lives of patients with chronic myeloid leukaemia (CML). CML is a disease of the myeloid stem cell characterized by marked splenomegaly and an increase in the production of white cells. The natural course of CML is a chronic phase, as described above, moving into an accelerated or blast crisis that, untreated, leads to death in a matter of weeks. Treatment aims at controlling the white blood cell count with splenectomy and the chemotherapy drugs busulfan, hydroxyurea or interferon. These measures can control the disease for a number of years. Bone marrow transplantation provides the only chance of cure, but only 20% of CML patients are suitable for this highly toxic treatment. Since the development and clinical use of imatinib mesylate, treatment approaches have changed. Traditional chemotherapy aimed at killing the mutant cancer cells; bone marrow transplantation cured 'by replacing the blood making cells'; now imatinib mesylate targets and blocks the *cause* of CML.

Where Did it all Begin?

The story began 40 years ago, in the 1960s. Researchers in Philadelphia were able to identify a common genetic mutation in patients with CML. Chromosome 22

Table 11.2   Anti-angiogenesis: Mode of Action

	Direct action	Indirect action
Target cell	Endothelial cell	Tumour cell
Effect	Prolonged use as a result of little or no drug resistance	Resistance possible caused by tumour cell mutation
Example	Endostatin	Herceptin

had a 'bit' missing. This became known as the Philadelphia chromosome and was found in 95% of CML patients. It was the first time that a genetic abnormality had been linked to a specific cancer. It took a further 13 years to find the 'missing bit', which had moved to chromosome 9. This phenomenon of moving from one chromosome to another is known as 'translocation'. The Philadelphia chromosome was a translocation from chromosome 22 to chromosome 9. This phenomenon had never been observed before. Since then, many other translocations have been detected.

The next chapter of the CML story was the identification of a rogue enzyme produced by the Philadelphia chromosome, known as Bcr-Abl. This enzyme changes a cell's activity and causes the cell to go into mass production, the characteristic of CML. The high white cell count seen in a peripheral blood count is a result of this enzyme switching on the mass production button. Scientists knew the genetic mutation for CML and had identified the single enzyme that switches on mass production. This left a clear direction for laboratory research to proceed in order to have an impact on the patient outcome and demonstrate true translational oncology research, namely:

Block Bcr-Abl — Block overproduction — Control/cure disease.

This challenge was taken up and in 1995 scientists had developed a potent specific inhibitor of Bcr-Abl. Preclinical work was encouraging and in the laboratory the inhibitor (now known as imatinib) did not demonstrate significant activity against normal cells, in stark contrast to traditional chemotherapy treatment. Clinical trials began in 1998, when 31 patients were entered into a trial using imatinib. All 31 had a complete haematological response to treatment and one third had a cytogenetic response, that is elimination of the Philadelphia chromosome. Phase 2 trials were initiated and produced the same exceptional results. In addition, imatinib was well tolerated and had very few side effects. Again the improved patient outcomes were a direct result of the collaboration of laboratory scientists and clinical staff, not forgetting the pioneering and brave patients.

The continued success of imatinib in the treatment of CML is one of the major breakthroughs in cancer care over the past decade. However, the story, although dramatic, is incomplete. Imatinib resistance has now occurred in some patients and a dermatological side effect has emerged. Very recently, a further, more serious concern has emerged, that of cardiac dysfunction. A very recent paper describes the development of significant ventricular ejection fraction reduction in 10 patients receiving imatinib (Kerkela et al., 2006). This adverse result is published alongside a report that imatinib affects the cardiac cells in mice and rats. The authors hypothesize the development of cardiac dysfunction may be related to the inhibition of the Abl kinase, which triggers the stress response in cardiomyocytes and induces cell death. This gives obvious cause for concern and dictates the research agenda: for scientists, to find out why; and for clinicians, to be cautious about who receives the drug and vigilant in observing patients already on imatinib. Angiogenesis research and the imatinib story, although different, are clear examples of scientists and clinicians working together with the same aim — better patient outcome.

Things don't always go so well, however. A recent event has dented some clinical research: a phase 1 clinical trial of a new drug went disastrously wrong. TGN1412 was developed to treat chronic inflammatory conditions, including rheumatoid arthritis, leukaemia and multiple sclerosis. Six healthy volunteers developed multi-organ failure following administration of the drug. Previous tests on animals showed no adverse events. Experts described the incident as unprecedented: 'This is an absolutely exceptional occurrence – I cannot remember anything comparable' (www.bbcnews.co.uk/1/hi/London/England).

The incident did of course give the scientists plenty to take back to the bench. The investigation suggests the event occurred because the human subjects' memory T-cells lost their sense of direction and started migrating into several areas of the body where they were not supposed to go, causing great damage (www.eurekalert.org.pubrelease).

The researchers retested memory T-cells in which TGN1412 had been previously stimulated, and injected them into healthy mice. These cells immediately migrated from the blood into many organs including the kidney, the heart and the gut, where they are not normally found unless there is an infection. In effect, this resulted in the body's immune system attacking itself. The whole event was true translational research. The new drug was developed by the scientists, tested by the clinicians, and the results were sent back to the scientists.

CONCLUSION

The coordinated approach now being taken to translational oncology research shows the commitment from both the laboratory and clinical fields to improving outcomes.

This can only be of huge benefit to patients, but is the NHS ready for their findings?

- Can the NHS cope with individualized treatments for patients?
- Can expertise be sustained?
- Can multidisciplinary teams cope with the time and effort involved in individualizing treatment en masse?
- Are hospital-based laboratories equipped for new technology?
- Can the health economy sustain new treatments?
- Are there any savings for the health economy from improved outcomes?
- Will there be any delay in starting treatment while refining individual plans?
- Are patients willing to wait for treatment?

These are real issues the NHS must face. Translational oncology research offers a fantastic opportunity to get research and clinical experts working together to improve outcomes for patients, but at a financial cost. Time will tell if we as a society can afford the price tag.

12 The Application of Research Methodology to Cancer Research

CARMEL SHEPPARD

The focus on the impressive list of advancements in the science of medicine leads us to sometimes neglect the art of medicine and potential for patients to feel somewhat dehumanized with 'high tech' medicine. Patients complain increasingly that 'high tech' medicine dehumanizes them. In the eternal quest for a new and better treatment for every known ailment, we have started to forget the other important needs of sick people (Fallowfield, 1990, p. 16).

The preceding chapters of this book have focused principally on the 'scientific' advances in cancer treatment, which have been primarily led by scientists and consequently mostly lie within the biomedical domain. This never-ending search for a greater understanding of what causes cancer, the biological effects of cancer on the body and new drug regimens to improve survival or even cure cancer, is essential and gives hope to us all. Indeed, the recent improvements in cancer survival rates demonstrate the advances made through such clinical research. Many patients' lives have been extended and enhanced through the introduction of new treatment regimens. Nevertheless, it is important not to forget the individual in all of this, who has to cope with the consequences of treatment, and live with the knowledge of a life-threatening illness and the devastating psychological effects that this brings to patient and family. In the past decade, it has been encouraging to see this aspect of care incorporated into many national clinical trials. There is growing recognition of its importance. This is illustrated by the emergence of quality of life as a required endpoint of many trials. However, although some progress has been made overall, there remains a paucity of nursing research to support certain nursing interventions, for example the advantages of specialist nursing intervention, as well as evidence relating to survivorship and rehabilitation and the relationship between nursing and patient outcomes (Corner, 2002; Richardson, Miller and Potter, 2002). Molassiotis *et al.* (2006) suggest that although symptoms are a common focus for research, little attention is paid to symptom management.

Following a literature review between 1980 and 2000, only 446 articles pertaining to cancer nursing research were identified, with less than 50% of these reporting primary nursing research (Richardson, Miller and Potter, 2002). A further systematic review of research relating to cancer nursing highlighted 619 papers published

The Biology of Cancer, Second Edition. Edited by J. Gabriel
© 2007 John Wiley & Sons, Ltd.

between 1994 and 2003, with only 18% of these papers originating from the United Kingdom (Molassiotis *et al.*, 2006). Interestingly, Molassiotis *et al.* (2006) and Murphy and Cowman (2006) also draw attention to the lack of multidisciplinary research. Acknowledging the importance of multidisciplinary care in relation to improved patient outcomes, collaborative research should be considered a key priority for the future, enabling us to explore and deliver optimum care regardless of professional boundaries.

Why do we need to continue to develop a research-based knowledge in cancer nursing? Research is the means through which we can gain a deeper understanding of the effects of cancer, formulate questions about patient care, test the effectiveness of pre-existing treatment and care, and in turn generate new ideas and evidence for practice. Understanding the effects of cancer and its physical and psychological impact will inevitably enable nursing to prepare patients more readily and support different patients experiencing similar circumstances. Ultimately, through research we aim to improve the overall quality of care for patients. In addition, we can strengthen the ability and opportunities for nurses to influence health-care policy by identifying the priorities and requirements of the future health service (DoH, 2000c). Sadly, the ability to do this has been hampered by the lack of research-based knowledge from which to draw, in comparison to our medical colleagues. It is not therefore surprising that health-care policy has traditionally been dominated by medicine. To ensure that patients benefit from a truly multidisciplinary approach to care, it is essential that we strive to develop this knowledge base. To do so is dependent not only on time and funding, but also on the ability to produce well-designed research that generates meaningful results.

The need to provide support for research within the NHS is now recognized by the Department of Health and outlined in the *Best Research for Best Health* document (DoH, 2006), which summarizes the need to support individuals conducting leading edge research, with the aim of having more patients and health professionals participating in research and ultimately improving health. In addition, major funding bodies of research, including government, charity and industry sectors, have come together to form a partnership through the National Cancer Research Institute (NCRI) to oversea cancer research in the United Kingdom. This organization focuses on the identification of gaps in research, opportunities for research, as well as funding support, with the aim of doubling the number of cancer patients entered into clinical trials (NCRI, 2004). Richardson, Miller and Potter (2002, p. 7) suggest that 'nursing research has too often been hampered by a limited focus, small sample sizes or inadequate rigour'. Poor quality research, particularly in relation to the lack of detail published, is further evidenced by Molassiotis *et al.* (2006) in a systematic review of worldwide cancer nursing research.

Although nurse education now includes training in research methodology, this has not always been the case, and the general prevailing culture in nursing outside academic institutions does not appear to sustain a major commitment to research. Richardson, Miller and Potter (2002) found that less than half (44%) of lead cancer nurses identified current nursing research initiatives in their clinical areas.

The Department of Health document *The Nursing Contribution to Cancer Care* (DoH, 2000d) suggests that one of the main barriers to research is the lack of training in this area. One of the functions of this chapter is to provide the reader with a basic understanding of research design, setting out steps towards developing a research proposal. It also aims to be a useful guide to critiquing published research.

Research is sometimes viewed as a series of complex methodological investigations reserved for academics, yet as nurses we are frequently engaged in research without realizing it. Research questions should be formulated within clinical practice, for example where there is limited evidence to support a particular aspect of clinical care, or through the observation of certain trends while working with a group of patients, or where there are concerns relating to treatments. Some clinical areas have developed journal clubs, which serve as a vehicle by which debate can be encouraged and ideas generated for investigation.

A well-structured proposal is a prerequisite for any research investigation. This should follow a systematic set of rules, which importantly demonstrate that rigour has been applied to the study. A research proposal should include a literature review that justifies the need for research in the given area. The overall aims and objectives of the project should be stated and, if the project aims to test theory (deduction), the hypothesis should be given. The design of the study, the sample unit, methods of data collection and analysis should be presented and justified. In developing a study, several considerations should be made:

- What is the topic to be investigated? This should be clear, focused on a specific aspect, free of ambiguity and achievable.
- What sort of information is needed before the start of the research, that is, literature search, anecdotal evidence?
- What sort of evidence is needed to answer the question?
- What type of investigation would provide the evidence needed?
- What are the resources required for the study, for example, time, finances, supervision and so on?
- What is a realistic time frame for the study?
- How will the results be disseminated?

The design of the study should be that which answers the question best. In reality, the design is often determined not only by the question but also by the underlying philosophical assumptions/perspectives of the researcher, which fall into either positivist or naturalistic perspectives, sometimes referred to as quantitative and qualitative research, respectively. Costs, time and expertise will also to some extent influence the design of the study.

QUANTITATIVE RESEARCH

Biomedical research is dominated by quantitative research, drawing from the positivist paradigm (Black, 1994); the underlying philosophical principle is that all human behaviour occurs through external stimuli, which can be observed and measured. A phenomenon is usually measured through quantitative research, which begins via the generation of ideas about the phenomenon of interest and subsequently develops ways to support or reject the hypothesis created. This form of research is particularly useful in gaining information about the effectiveness of treatment and patient outcomes in response to treatment in terms of generalized numerical data, and hence differs from the qualitative approach, which focuses on the subjective experiences of individuals.

Sample sizes should be stated in the proposal. In quantitative research, sample size is generally calculated at the outset of the study, and this is essential if the researcher wishes to have a high chance of detecting any statistically significant effect. It is advisable to seek advice from a statistician when calculating sample size. The researcher attempts to demonstrate that the difference between any two groups relates to the treatment or what is being tested, and nothing else. As we can never be absolutely sure that what is observed relates only to what is being tested, the significance level (p value) is generally set at between 0.01 and 0.05 (i.e. a 1–5% chance that the differences were not caused by the hypothesis) and is determined by the researcher. The level of significance is the degree of risk that the researcher is willing to take that they will reject a null hypothesis when it is really true, otherwise known as a type I error. A type II error is when the researcher mistakenly accepts a false null hypothesis. Samples that are too small have a high risk of failing to demonstrate a real difference. Some academic journals now decline publication of data from small studies unless other sources of information published in the related field are limited. Importantly, if statistical power is low, the results of the study may be heavily criticized – 'statistical power is a measure of how likely the study is to produce a statistically significant result for a difference between groups of a given magnitude (i.e. the ability to detect a true difference)' (Bowling, 1997, p. 149). It is normally accepted that the power of a study should be between 80% and 90% (i.e. you have an 80–90% chance of detecting a statistically significant result) (Bowling 1997; Salkind, 2000; Greenhalgh, 2001).

A further consideration is the sampling method, which should avoid unwanted bias and ensure that the sample is representative of the particular patients under investigation. There are basically two types of sampling you can include: probability and non-probability sampling; in quantitative research the main aim of the study is to ensure representation of the target population, so probability sampling is the preferred method. There is a variety of approaches to probability sampling, including simple random sampling, systematic random sampling, stratified random sampling and cluster sampling, which are described further by Bowling (1997) (Table 12.1).

When designing a study, the researcher must consider the tools of measurement that can be varied, for example, patient satisfaction may be measured by postal questionnaire, structured or semi-structured interviews, or telephone interviews. Justification of the methods used should be stated in the proposal. Issues such as cost, increasing the opportunity for greater response rates and convenience for the patient will usually influence the decision concerning how data will be collected. If

Table 12.1 Randomization sampling frames

Simple random sampling	Each participant has an equal chance of being selected for either the control or experimental group.
Stratified random sampling	If the sampling frame contains a large variation in variables, for example, age, disease site and so on, the researcher may wish to ensure that the sample is representative. According to the variables, units in the sample frame are separated into strata (layers) and samples are drawn from each stratum.
Cluster sampling	Units are divided into groups, which are subsequently sampled randomly (usually used for economic purposes). Again there may be difficulties with clusters being unrepresentative, for example participants from a shared environment may not be truly reflective of the total population.
Systematic sampling	Units are selected at intervals from lists, for example, every fifth patient on the list. The researcher should be aware however of the potential bias that lists may have.

a questionnaire is used, care should be taken in the design to ensure that participants can clearly understand what is requested of them, that it is presented in such a manner as to encourage completion and that it is free from ambiguity, all of which may affect the ability to analyse the results. Issues of confidentiality should also be considered so that participants' answers are not influenced by the possibility of being identified. A pilot study should be undertaken to test the questionnaire and confirm that the questions measure what they are intended to measure before large-scale implementation in the final study.

One of the increasing areas of investigation is patient based outcomes. Measurements of quality of life, psychological morbidity and attitude tend to be complex and any measurement tool should be tested for both reliability and validity. Reliability is the extent to which the instrument demonstrates reproducibility and consistency through repeated administration (Bowling, 1997). 'Validity is an assessment of whether an instrument measures what it aims to measure' (Bowling, 1997, p. 130). Numerous tools have already been developed and tested, for example the General Health Questionnaire (Goldberg and Williams, 1988) and the Hospital Anxiety and Depression Scale (HAD) (Zigmond and Snaith, 1983), both of which measure psychological morbidity. Quality-of-life tools are also available (Bowling, 2001), some of which have been specifically designed for studies relating to cancer, such as the Functional Assessment of Cancer Therapy (Cella *et al.,* 1993) and the EORTC Quality of Life Questionnaire (Sprangers *et al.,* 1993). Other measurements may include service outcomes, cost-effectiveness and clinical outcome measures, for example numbers of tumours detected or recurrence of tumour, which may be collected either retrospectively or prospectively from the patients' medical/nursing notes.

Generally, quantitative research produces large quantities of numerical data that are presented either in descriptive form (data that describe the characteristics of a sample or population) or as inferential statistics (data that enable inferences from the sample data to be applied to a population) (Salkind, 2000). How the results are to be analysed and presented should be considered in the proposal and design of the study.

While there is a variety of approaches to quantitative research, three main designs are described below, although these should not be viewed as exhaustive of quantitative designs.

RANDOMIZED CONTROLLED TRIALS

The randomized controlled trial (RCT) is generally referred to as the gold standard of research and is often used to compare interventions. It is basically an experimental trial comparing two or more groups of patients who are randomly allocated to either one form of treatment or another. Through this random allocation, the risk of extraneous variables is reduced, thus increasing the chance that any changes are caused only by the intervention, so allowing the cause and effect to be determined. The essential characteristics of this design include a hypothesis that one form of treatment or intervention will cause a particular effect (e.g. the nurse may develop a hypothesis that wound healing is improved with the use of a particular dressing and then aim to test this hypothesis). The study is prospective in nature and patients are randomly allocated to receive either the intervention (e.g. the dressing to be tested) or the control (which in this case would be the accepted standard form of dressing). The researcher attempts to eradicate bias through the randomization process and thus compare two groups that are very similar apart from the variable under investigation (Figure 12.1).

As well as investigating the effects of certain types of intervention, drug or procedure, the RCT is also useful in determining the most appropriate provision of care. RCTs are not appropriate for studies where there is difficulty in randomization, for example it would be unethical to randomize patients into different arms of treatment when one treatment is known to have superiority.

There are some variations of RCT design, an example of which is the simple crossover method. This allows both groups to act as their own control by exposing them sequentially to both arms of the study. However, this would not be suitable for conditions that fluctuate before treatment or if there was the possibility of residual effects of the first arm of the treatment causing potential bias (Bowling, 1997).

Example of RCT (Baildam *et al.*, 2001)

Objective

To compare nurse-led versus doctor-led follow-up after a diagnosis of breast cancer and completion of treatment.

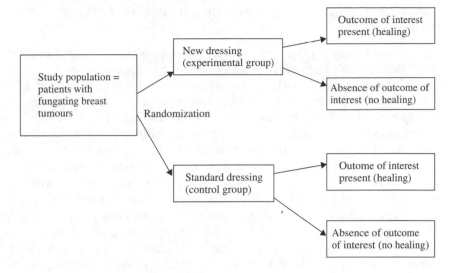

Figure 12.1   Basic design structure for randomized controlled trials (RCTs).

Design

After a diagnosis of breast cancer, patients are generally followed up by the consultant and their team for a period of 5−10 years. This randomized study compared follow-up by two specially trained, experienced specialist nurses (experimental group) with the traditional follow-up by doctors (control group).

Sample Size

525 patients were randomized to each of the groups.

Outcome Measures

These included differences in detection of recurrence between the two groups, recognition of patient psychological morbidity and patient satisfaction between the two groups. Psychological morbidity was measured using well-validated measurement tools, including HAD and the Spielberger State Anxiety. Satisfaction was also measured, using the Fallowfield Satisfaction with Consultation Questionnaire.

Results

The results demonstrated that nurse recognition of psychological morbidity was greater than that recorded by doctors. No differences in the ability to detect recurrence were found. The authors conclude that nurse-led clinics can provide high-quality care equal at least to that of their medical equivalents.

QUASI-EXPERIMENTS: CASE–CONTROL STUDIES AND COHORT STUDIES

A case–control study may be used to investigate a problem related to a cause of disease. Patients with a particular condition (cases) are compared with an identical group of individuals who do not have the condition (controls). Both groups should be identically matched except for the condition under study. Case–control studies are generally retrospective, and accounts of past history and exposure are investigated to ascertain the common lifetime exposures, linking these to possible causation of disease. The benefits of this form of research are that the researcher can study multiple exposures and diseases that have long latent periods, for example breast cancer may recur after some 15–20 years, hence the effects of breast screening should be evaluated over this period. A case–control study is also useful in situations where it would be unethical to carry out an experimental study or where little is known about the cause of the disease. The evidence gained from this sort of research is generally considered lower down the ladder than that from the RCT. There is potential to overlook influencing factors that are outside the realms of the study, and thus the results may be less reliable.

There may also be difficulties with selection bias, particularly as the researcher must attempt to rule out other possible threats to the validity of the findings, such as other exposures. Information bias is also a potential problem because exposure status is determined after the outcome has occurred and therefore participants' recall of exposure may be blurred.

Example of Case–Control (Draper *et al.*, 1997)

Objective

To test the hypothesis that 'childhood leukaemia and non-Hodgkin's lymphoma can be caused by fathers' exposure to ionizing radiation before the conception of the child, and more generally, to investigate whether such radiation exposure of either patient is a cause of childhood cancer'.

Design

The case group (35 949 children diagnosed with cancer) was compared with the control group (a group of individuals selected from the birth register for the same area of birth, matched on sex and born within 6 months of the case).

Outcome Measures

These included (i) parental employment as radiation worker before conception of child, (ii) cumulative dose of external ionizing radiation for various periods of employment before conception of child and (iii) dose during pregnancy.

Results

Although the researchers confirmed that the fathers of the children with leukaemia or non-Hodgkin's lymphoma were significantly more likely than the fathers of the controls to have been radiation workers, they concluded that this did not relate to a preconceived radiation dose. As such, the absence of a relationship between dose and risk led the researchers to believe that these findings may be related either to chance or perhaps to some characteristic other than exposure to radiation.

COHORT STUDIES

Cohort studies can be prospective or retrospective (historical) depending on the time that the exposure data were measured. The essential feature of all cohort studies is that the exposure is measured before outcome (Greenhalgh, 2001). In a prospective cohort study, the researcher begins with individuals who have not yet had the outcome of interest (e.g. bowel cancer) and follow the group forward in time measuring exposure (e.g. diet) to see if the outcome of interest occurs (e.g. bowel cancer diagnosis). In a retrospective cohort study, exposure is measured using data collected before the study started (e.g. by looking back through case notes at the main exposures during the study period), although recall bias may be an issue with retrospective data. In addition to bias, Brennan and Croft (1994) highlight the importance of confounding, which must be considered in any cohort study. Unlike the RCT, in which participants are randomly allocated to either the experimental or the control arm, participants of cohort studies choose to be exposed or not and this in itself may affect the outcomes of both groups. 'As a consequence, if a confounder is not recognized and adjustments made for its effect the exposed and unexposed groups in such studies will not be comparable' (Brennan and Croft, 1994). Figure 12.2 shows a cohort study design.

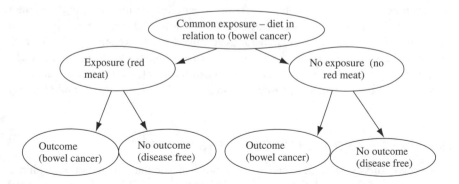

Figure 12.2   Cohort study design.

Example of a Cohort Study (Graham *et al.*, 2002)

Objective

To confirm the relationship between severely stressful life experiences and relapse of breast cancer found in a previous case–control study.

Design

This was a prospective study recruiting a cohort of women newly diagnosed with breast cancer. The researchers controlled the group for a biological prognostic factor (i.e. other factors that might affect recurrence rates such as lymph node status and tumour grade).

Outcome Measure

Recurrence of disease.

Data Collection

Women were interviewed every 18 months over a period of 5 years, collecting data on stressful experiences and depression (including data on experiences 12 months before diagnosis).

Results

Overall, the researchers found no increased risk of recurrence in women who had one or more severely stressful life experiences in the year before diagnosis compared with women who did not, and of those who had had stressful experiences since diagnosis the results demonstrated a lower risk of recurrence, confirming that stressful events did not lead to increased risk of recurrence.

The interesting thing about this study is that it is a good example of how different designs may affect research outcome. As the researchers themselves point out, their findings differ from those in an earlier study (Ramirez *et al.*, 1989) which used case–control methods. The researchers suggest that this may relate to problems with retrospective studies, such as the difficulty of recalling stressful experiences and the possibility that patients look back for something to blame for the development of recurrence; they suggest a prospective study enables greater recall and accuracy of data.

DESCRIPTIVE AND ANALYTIC SURVEYS

Descriptive surveys are designed to measure a particular phenomenon within a cross-section of the population, for example in cancer care this design may be used to identify the prevalence of cervical cancer in the Jewish population, or perhaps the prevalence of cervical cancer in women who have had numerous sexual partners. Consequently surveys are retrospective and can be used to generate a hypothesis or test a hypothesis, for example that cervical cancer is more common among women with multiple sexual relationships. The benefits are that large numbers of people can be surveyed, although, as with any retrospective data, recall may add bias. In addition, surveys cannot be used to indicate a direction of cause.

Analytic surveys are longitudinal and record data at frequent intervals, making this approach useful in monitoring the effects of interventions, for example health promotion activities, through observation of changes in lifestyle patterns. One of the difficulties is the possibility of sample attrition, and the prospective approach means that results can take time and tend to be expensive, particularly in relation to administration costs. Furthermore, in both these designs survey information tends to be superficial, and breadth rather than depth is emphasized (LoBiondo-Wood and Haber, 1998).

QUALITATIVE RESEARCH

The naturalistic approach differs in its underlying philosophical beliefs in that it is based on the idea that there is no objective reality but that we all develop our own subjective reality; hence there is an increased focus on feelings, experiences, thoughts and interactions. Originating from social scientists, the naturalist research approach, often referred to as qualitative research, is concerned with the development of theory (induction) rather than the testing of theory (deduction). Acceptance and value recognition of qualitative research in medicine have been somewhat slow, although in recent years there has been increasing publication of qualitative research in highly regarded medical science literature, suggesting a shift in acknowledgement and appreciation of what qualitative research may convey.

The strength of quantitative research lies in its ability to produce large-scale data, which can be tested for reliability and validity, and consequently can be generalized to a number of settings. The strength of qualitative research lies in its intimacy with the truth and its ability to explore depths of meanings (Greenhalgh, 2001). In contrast to quantitative research, rather than focusing on a single aspect of measurement, whereby certain elements of depth may be lost, qualitative research illuminates the experience in an attempt to understand its depth. In nursing, much of the published research lies within this paradigm, perhaps because nursing itself is concerned more with a holistic approach to individualized patient-centred care (Munhall, 1982). It is important to recognize, however, the limitations of knowledge based entirely on small-scale, non-generalizable studies, and there have been calls for a move towards an eclectic approach.

In contrast to experimental research, which tends to produce large-scale and often depersonalized data (Parahoo, 1997, p. 209), the numbers of participants are generally kept small, with the concern being more the depth and richness of information than the quantity of participants and statistical power.

Informants/participants are usually selected on the basis that they have experienced the phenomenon under investigation and are thus more able to shed light on it, rather than the random or representative sample needed within quantitative studies. Sampling methods include purposive/theoretical sampling, convenience/opportunistic sampling and snowballing (Table 12.2). As a result of the small size of the sample, it is important to recognize the limitations in terms of generalizability to other settings and patients.

Qualitative research is particularly useful where there is no prior knowledge and a need to generate theory; hence research using a qualitative approach will generally begin with a broad topic of investigation and, as the research progresses, the researcher will narrow the focus of research as the phenomenon is uncovered. Popay and Williams (1998, p. 34) describe qualitative research as 'focusing on the meanings that people attach to experience, the relationship between knowledge, experience and action and the social factors that shape these processes'. Within qualitative research, the uniqueness of individuals is expressed and the researcher seeks to uncover and understand this uniqueness through immersion in the social context. Critics might argue that, through this immersion, qualitative researchers fail to recognize the impact that they themselves have on the participants. Consequently, the researcher must constantly be aware of the possible influences of researcher bias and remain neutral. It is important to recognize that qualitative research is often criticized for its subjectivity and lack of scientific rigour; hence it is particularly important to pay attention to research design and method of data collection and analysis, and to provide sufficient detail to enable external assessment by others. Indeed, Koch (1996, p. 177) suggests that the resolution of issues of rigour should be the 'current pre-occupation' for qualitative researchers.

Data collection methods are generally guided by the question, the philosophical framework and the principles adopted by the researcher. Most commonly, data collection occurs through either in-depth/unstructured interviews, semi-structured

Table 12.2   Sampling methods for qualitative research

Purposive sampling/Theoretical sampling	The researcher deliberately chooses the sample on the basis of known characteristics. For example, patients may be selected on the basis that they have experienced a certain phenomenon and thus can provide insight to the investigation. Theoretical sampling continues according to the data generated, searching for new data to develop the theory until no new data emerge.
Convenience/Opportunistic sampling	The researcher chooses the sample simply as the opportunity presents itself, for example, easy to recruit, likely to want to participate.
Snowball sampling	Arises from convenience sampling but gathers further participants through introduction to others known to the original sample who are also in the group of interest.

interviews, observation and field notes, focus groups, diaries or examination of documentation. To capture the entirety of the data during interviews, the researcher generally tape-records the participant sessions. The enormity of the data recorded should not be underestimated as the volumes of data will take considerable time to transcribe and analyse. A 1-hour interview can take 2−4 hours to transcribe.

Analysis of the data usually follows a step-by-step approach, which generally involves the identification of themes and categories. Various techniques for data analysis have been described (Colaizzi 1978; Van Manen, 1990). Computer software is available to assist in the analysis of the contents of transcripts, such as NUD.IST (Richards and Richards, 1990). As mentioned earlier, one of the main criticisms of qualitative research is the lack of attention to rigour during the data collection and analysis phases. The researcher should seek to enhance the reliability of the data through the involvement of independent assessors, ensuring that the researcher has not overinterpreted or misinterpreted data. Validation strategies sometimes involve checking back with the participants to confirm with them that the themes reflect their experiences and interpretations (Mays and Pope, 1995), although O'Mahony (2001) highlights the potential difficulties with this, particularly if the participants have revealed difficult, painful memories; therefore this should be carefully planned.

Final presentation of the data should be considered. The themes or categories should be exhibited with accompanying text examples demonstrating how they were developed and how the associated meanings or interpretations were attained. Data should be presented authentically. The reader should be able to follow the decision pathways and interpretations of the researcher so that they can assess the trustworthiness of the data.

As with quantitative research, there is a variety of different approaches/ philosophical underpinnings to qualitative research. Three approaches are demonstrated below, although these by no means describe the full diversity of qualitative methods.

GROUNDED THEORY

This was developed and described by Glaser and Strauss (1967). Grounded theorists search to uncover the 'social processes present in human interaction' (Cutliffe, 2000). Where there is little known about particular phenomena or processes, grounded theory enables the development of a theory and goes beyond the mere description of a situation. Theoretical development occurs through constant comparison of data and is characterized by a non-linear process in which the researcher constantly revisits the data for comparatives, differences, similarities and patterns; hence data collection and analysis usually occur simultaneously. Unlike the unstructured interview process in phenomenology, the researcher using grounded theory will often adopt a variety of data collection methods to ensure that the study is grounded in facts (Wimpenny and Gass, 2000). Data collection continues until completely saturated, with no new concepts/categories emerging, so there are no limitations to the number of participants. Sampling is motivated by the emerging theory, hence 'theoretical sampling' (Cutliffe, 2000), rather than the 'purposeful' sampling usually used in phenomenology — although most researchers presently use the terms 'theoretical' and 'purposeful' interchangeably, leading to some confusion for the reader. Several authors have discussed and highlighted the difficulties with method slurring, which is not uncommon within the literature (Baker, Wuest and Norager-Stern, 1992; Wimpenny and Gass, 2000).

Example of Grounded Theory (Thomas and Retsas, 1999)

Purpose of the Study

To construct a grounded theory that explains how the spirituality of people with terminal cancer develops as they make sense of and come to terms with their diagnosis.

Sample

Nineteen patients were purposively sampled, selected on the basis that they could provide insight into the phenomena being studied. The sample was developed by 'snowballing', for example by one person introducing another to the study.

Data Collection

In-depth interviews, with guided questions that were modified during the course of the data collection. Follow-up interviews were conducted to debrief the participants and clarify data and insights.

Analysis

Constant comparative method of analysis described by Strauss and Corbin (1990).

Findings

This study found that people with terminal cancer develop a sense of spirituality as they make sense of and come to terms with their diagnosis. In seeking self-preservation, three interconnected behaviours were identified, that is 'taking it all in', 'getting on with it' and 'putting it all together'. 'Taking it all in' involved the response to and questioning of the diagnosis. 'Getting on with it' was when the participants were more able to confront the reality of their diagnosis and when they began to confront their cancer and mobilize by connecting with self, others, God or a higher being. 'Putting it all together' reflected how participants created meaning in their terminal cancer and began to discover their 'self', taking stock of their life, changing their outlook, transforming, becoming spiritual and expanding their consciousness.

Learning

Transacting self-preservation is made complete as the person reaches a deeper level of understanding of self that is imbued with spiritual growth. It gives deep meaning and richness to the person's life as he or she transcends everyday experiences in the journey to death. The authors suggest that nurses must recognize that people with terminal cancer need help to find spiritual meaning. They suggest that nurses' 'spiritual support may mean nothing more than taking the time to provide physical and psychological caring that touches the spirit'. They highlight the fact that some patients may find it difficult to articulate their spirituality.

PHENOMENOLOGY

Since the late 1980s there has been increasing interest in the use of phenomenological research published within the nursing literature; however, varied interpretations of the original philosophical assumptions underpinning this approach have led to much criticism (Koch, 1995; Paley, 1997; Van der Zalm and Bergum, 2000).

Phenomenology as described by Husserl (1859–1938) is the study of the 'lived experience', whereby the researcher aims to uncover or illuminate the real meaning of human lived experience by asking questions such as 'can you tell me what it is like to have been given a diagnosis of cancer?' In Husserlian phenomenology, importantly, the researcher aims to 'bracket' any of their own preconceptions in an attempt truly to reflect and describe the world as viewed by the participant. Koch (1996, p. 176) suggests that 'the hallmark of any genuinely phenomenological inquiry is that its task is a matter of describing'. Heidegger, a student of Husserl, later developed Husserl's original concepts, placing greater importance on understanding the 'meanings' attached to the experience of individuals. He rejected the notion of 'bracketting', suggesting that one cannot separate the description from one's own interpretation of it and hence, during data analysis, the prior experiences of the researcher are merged with the participant's data (Koch, 1996).

The primary objective of phenomenological research is to describe and provide an understanding of a person's lived experience: 'instead of pin-pointing a minute segment of experience as in quantitative research, the phenomenological view enlarges the experience and attempts to understand it in the complexity of its context' (Thibodeau and MacRae, 1997). This is done through the use of in-depth interviews, with the overall purpose of the data analysis process being to maintain the original meaning and demonstrate rigour. Crist and Tanner (2003) provide a guide to analysing interviews and observations, as well as dealing with issues such as question development and sampling issues.

Example of a Phenomenological Study (Breaden, 1997)

Purpose

Using hermeneutic phenomenology, this study examined the experiences of women who had finished treatment and were at least 8 months post-cancer diagnosis.

Sample Size

Six women.

Data Collection

In-depth interviews, each lasting approximately an hour.

Analysis

After analysis of transcripts from in-depth interviews, return visits were made to the participants to discuss individual transcripts. Using the process of thematic analysis described by Van Manen (1990), the transcripts were read and reread several times to get a sense of the whole. This occurred during ongoing data collection in order to enable the researcher to ask more focused questions. A highlighting approach was used to isolate thematic statements. Statements relating to the experience of surviving cancer were isolated and recurring themes were identified.

Issues of Rigour

The participants were revisited for clarification of meanings. Dependability and confirmability were attempted through the use of a reflective journal.

Findings

Original text was used to demonstrate the construction of themes. Women describe a survival process that includes 'feeling whole again', 'the body as a house of suspicion', 'the future in question', 'changes in time', 'lucky to be alive' and 'sharing the journey'.

Comments

Although the researcher suggests that data analysis occurred simultaneously with data collection to enable the asking of more focused questions, arguably in keeping with phenomenological principles interviews are generally unstructured, for example Koch (1996, p. 1979) states: 'I do not ask specific questions; the exchange is entirely open'. Despite keeping a reflective journal, it is unclear from the publication how this information was used and how it informed the analysis process, which would have been helpful to ascertain the trustworthiness of the data.

ETHNOGRAPHY

The primary purpose of ethnographic studies is to understand human behaviour and its relationship to the culture and social context in which it occurs (Hammersley and Atkinson, 1983). Ethnography can be defined as the systematic process of observing, detailing, describing, documenting and analysing the behaviours of cultural groups. To do this, the researcher enters the world of the group of interest to see it through the eyes of the individuals within the culture, and uses various methods of data collection, which usually include participant field observation as well as face-to-face interviews and recording of interactive dialogue within the cultural setting. Analysis occurs simultaneously in field and involves the analysis of language, behaviour and field notes (Parahoo, 1997).

Example of an Ethnographic Study (Cope, 1995)

Purpose

To investigate the function of a breast cancer support group as perceived by the participants.

Sample

A convenience sample of 15 women diagnosed with breast cancer, all of whom were attending a cancer support group.

Data Collection

Participant observation, plus two key informant interviews to seek further clarification, explanation and validation of the data.

Analysis

Content analysis of audio-tape recordings from 10 meetings and from the two key informants. Credibility was addressed through validation of the data by the informants. Auditability/reliability was checked through an independent review of the analysis process by an experienced researcher.

Findings

Three major categories were formed, which described the purpose and benefits that the patients thought belonged to the group. These were exchanging information, sharing the illness experience and providing strength. All three categories were described by the researcher, and evidence was provided for each category.

Learning

Nurses should be cognizant of the functions of a breast cancer support group so that this information can be shared with patients.

CONCLUSION

Although this chapter has dedicated itself to an overview of research methodology, the effect of research on the patient should be given precedence. We must make sure that patients are well informed and safe, and that participation is voluntary (Entwistle, Tritter and Calnan, 2002). Any research that involves patients should have prior ethical committee approval. Madsen *et al.* (2002) and Cox (1999) highlight the complex psychological processes experienced by patients in decision-making about participation, particularly in relation to experimental treatments. One way of maximizing acceptability for patients is to involve them in the initial design, so that the patient perspective can be encompassed.

Many patients are asked to participate in national trials and as nurses we should endeavour to offer support and information to patients in their decision-making processes. Jenkins and Fallowfield (2000) report that less than 5% of patients are currently recruited to clinical trials in the United Kingdom. Naturally, if we are to advance knowledge about cancer treatments further, this figure must be improved. Jenkins and Fallowfield (2000) suggest that non-participation can be influenced by both the physician and the patient. It would not be surprising if nurses also played some part in influencing patients. Consequently, not only is there a need to have a basic understanding of research methodology, but also to keep up to date with the current clinical trials in our specialist areas.

In summary, research has a crucial part to play in the development of nursing care and treatment for patients with cancer. This chapter has outlined a range of methodological designs and, although quantitative and qualitative research have been presented independently of each other, there may be advantages in combining these methodological approaches. Sadly, in preparing this chapter there was much evidence of poorly designed nursing research with little attention to rigour within the literature. It is essential therefore that, if we are to gain recognition for our contribution to research and knowledge, we seek to redress this by ensuring that any research that we as nurses undertake is well designed to give meaningful results.

13 Research Ethics Relating to Cancer

DAVID CARPENTER

Research is surely a good thing; it is not immediately obvious that there are any ethical considerations beyond some sort of imperative to undertake it. After all, there would be no reliably effective treatment and care were it not for research and the evidence base of health-care interventions would simply not exist without it. Effective cancer care and treatment rely on previous and current research and we hope that future endeavours will provide hitherto elusive curative treatments for some of the most serious cancers. Although strongly supporting research, this chapter aims to elucidate necessary limits on the enterprise. These limits may be identified by considering issues such as the motives of the researcher, the value of the research and, most importantly, the welfare of the participants. In simple terms, these limits highlight the differences between research (which might none the less provide extremely useful knowledge) and *ethical* research.

Ethical research is, ideally, altruistically motivated and worth while, and ensures the welfare of participants. These ideals are seldom fully attainable. The purpose of ethical review of research proposals is to assess the degree to which they are compromised, and whether a proposed study falls within acceptable limits.

It is likely that many readers will be considering undertaking a research project, probably as part of undergraduate or postgraduate study. The primary purpose of such a study will be the award of a degree: hardly an altruistic motive. It is also highly likely that the project will be small scale, with little potential to provide any significant benefit to participants or others in the future. Although it may be unlikely that any participants will suffer significant harm, they will necessarily have to give their time and energy. To put the matter bluntly, students often *use* patients to gain a degree.

It is this issue of using people, albeit in the pursuit of valuable knowledge, that makes research ethically sensitive. Health-care research poses some of the greatest concerns, given that in most cases participants are sick, and in some cases they might be critically ill or dying. Cancer patients are often in these latter categories. Is it defensible to use them to gain knowledge, particularly when they, as participants, might gain little or no benefit and, indeed, might suffer considerable harm? Of

The Biology of Cancer, Second Edition. Edited by J. Gabriel
© 2007 John Wiley & Sons, Ltd.

course, the answer to this question is 'it all depends'. It depends on the skill of the researcher, the value of the research and the risks posed to the participants. Again, it is the purpose of ethical review to establish whether the proposed research satisfies this 'it all depends' criterion.

This chapter will consider research ethics from the perspectives of, first, the researcher, second, the research and, third, the participant. It will include an overview of the work of research ethics committees, particularly NHS Research Ethics Committees (NHSRECs), and their roles within the recently announced National Research Ethics Service (The Central Office for Research Ethics Committees (COREC, 2006)). Before embarking on this enterprise, however, it is worth reflecting on some historical and some surprisingly recent examples of unethical research.

UNETHICAL RESEARCH

Kennedy and Grubb (2000) suggest that the greatest incentive to regulate health-care research was awareness of the atrocities committed during the Second World War in the name of medical research. According to Evans and Evans (1996), 23 doctors were convicted at the Nuremberg trials. Their deeds included: freezing subjects in an attempt to discover the most effective means of treating hypothermia; deliberately infecting subjects with malaria with the aim of discovering suitable vaccines; and inflicting and subsequently infecting wounds to test the efficacy of sulfanilamide as an antibacterial agent. Not surprisingly, many of the subjects died; all suffered immeasurably. The research did, however, provide useful knowledge and the doctors were able to provide more effective treatment for German troops. It is a chilling fact that valuable knowledge can be obtained relatively easily if researchers have no concern for the welfare of their subjects.

The doctors concerned were found guilty of crimes against humanity, and of fundamental breaches of human rights. The Nuremberg Code followed, as an attempt to regulate future research on humans. The Nuremberg Code has been replaced by the World Medical Association's Declaration of Helsinki (2000), which remains a key regulator of medical research. International codes, declarations and treaties are typically used to protect human rights, but they necessarily require states to sign up to them in order to be effective. There is little to prevent the unethical researcher undertaking their investigations in non-subscribing countries, although they would certainly find difficulty publishing any results, valuable or otherwise. European citizens enjoy protection of fundamental human rights by virtue of the European Convention of Human Rights. The articles of the convention form part of the Human Rights Act 1998, which came into force in 2000. The rights of research participants are therefore protected by the duties of researchers, as stated in the Declaration of Helsinki, and by law. Further protection to research participants in clinical trials, particularly children and mentally incapacitated people, is provided through the Medicines for Human Use (Clinical Trials) Regulations 2004. This legislation came into place following implementation of the European Union Directive 2001/20/EC into UK law. It was the first piece of legislation, albeit secondary, to regulate some aspects of healthcare research. More recent primary legislation includes the Human Tissue Act 2004 and the Mental Capacity Act 2005; these will be discussed later in the chapter.

Despite the theoretical protection of research participants, there are more recent examples of unethical research, some of which triggered legal responses and associated reorganizations of NHSRECs. According to an urgent communication from the Chief Medical Officer of Health in 2000 (DoH, 2000f), volunteers who had taken part in trials at the Chemical and Biological Defence Establishment at Porton Down were to be offered a Medical Assessment Programme (MAP). This followed investigations by Wiltshire Constabulary after it received complaints from volunteers. It would appear that the volunteers were suffering unusual ill health, which they were attributing to their participation in the trials.

Between the 1940s and 1980s, some 20 000 servicemen volunteered to be exposed to low levels of mustard gas and nerve agents, including sarin. The communication reports the Ministry of Defence (MoD) as not having seen any evidence connecting ill health with participation in the trials. In July 2001 (Anon, 2001), the government launched an independent medical investigation. By this time there was compelling evidence that some volunteers had received dangerous doses and, moreover, some claimed to have been duped into believing that they would be researching the common cold.

A public outcry followed exposure of practices in Bristol and Alder Hey children's hospitals (DoH, 1999). Organs and tissues were routinely retained after post mortem examinations for several purposes, including medical research; it later became clear that no significant research was undertaken. Although in some cases parents had signed consent forms, it transpired that they were not made explicitly aware of the implications of doing so. After this exposure, the Chief Medical Officer of Health (CMO) conducted a census (DoH, 2000e) to establish the nature and volume of retained organs and tissues in NHS trusts and medical schools. Among his conclusions was recognition of the potential research value of organs and tissues from the dead, but he urged that this should not override the feelings of families and the need for informed consent.

A further outcry followed the discovery that 20 000 brains had been taken for research after post mortem examinations. An investigation was conducted by Her Majesty's Inspector of Anatomy, Dr Jeremy Metters, after Mrs Elaine Isaacs discovered that her late husband's brain had been removed post mortem and given to Manchester University for research, without her consent. The Isaacs Report (DoH, 2003b) revealed the extent of the practice. It is clear, then, that unethical research is not a matter to be consigned to distant history. Arguably the need for rigorous ethical review and monitoring has never been stronger.

THE RESEARCHER

Most health-care researchers are health-care professionals or at least working under their direction. This situation gives rise to an interesting analysis with regard to duty. It would seem obvious that health-care professionals, including nurses, have a primary duty towards the patient as an individual; any research activity is likely to subordinate this duty to the wider interests of a greater population. In simple terms, the role of the nurse changes from duty-bound practitioner to researcher.

In the introduction to the Code of Professional Conduct, the Nursing and Midwifery Council (NMC, 2004) states:

> As a registered nurse, midwife or health visitor you are personally accountable for your practice. In caring for patients and clients, you must:
>
> - Respect the patient or client as an individual
> - Obtain consent before you give any treatment or care
> - Protect confidential information
> - Cooperate with others in the team
> - Maintain your knowledge and competence
> - Be trustworthy
> - Act to identify and minimize any risks to patients and clients.

The NMC (2004) goes on to state: 'These are the shared values of all the United Kingdom health care regulatory bodies.' It is important that the professional imperatives stated above are described as 'values', had they been absolute duties most would be breached in the course of research. Most research entails using data gained from individuals or groups of patients to interrogate hypotheses or construct theories. The results of research can then be used to benefit the wider population. A health-care researcher simply cannot respect patients and clients *as individuals*.

Analysis of the list of values stated above raises some problems. If these values were viewed as absolute duties, there would be inevitable conflicts, for example it would be very difficult, if not impossible, to maintain knowledge and competence while continuing to respect patients as individuals. Equally it would be difficult to maintain knowledge and competence without accessing and analysing data that might otherwise be treated as confidential. The usual purpose of collecting confidential health-care data is to optimize individual care and treatment; using it in the context of research is clearly a departure from this primary purpose. How can these problems be solved? The short answer is that a complete solution is unlikely; however, acceptable compromises can result in ethical research. The nature of these compromises can be understood by investigating:

- The roles and duties of health-care practitioners
- The regulation of research activities
- The rights of participants.

The last two issues are addressed later; the first is dealt with in more detail at this stage.

Health-care regulatory bodies typically provide further guidance to practitioners with regard to research. The NMC (2006) has produced criteria for safe and ethical conduct of research, and states:

> You must always refer to the *Code of Professional Conduct*. This document provides the framework for all actions of registrants. As well as using these documents, you need to be sure that the research or clinical trial you are carrying out meets specific criteria. These are that:
>
> * the project must be approved by the LREC;
> * management approval must be gained where necessary;
> * arrangements for obtaining consent must be clearly understood by all those involved;
> * confidentiality must be maintained;
> * patients/clients must not be exposed to unacceptable risks;
> * patients/clients should be included in the development of proposed projects where appropriate;
> * accurate records must be kept and research questions need to be well structured and aimed at producing clearly anticipated care or service outcomes and benefits.

Given the overriding obligation to refer to the Code of Professional Conduct, it might be observed that the most compelling criteria are those requiring LREC (NHSREC) and management approval for research; these are considered later.

The duties of health-care practitioners are wider than those prescribed by health-care regulatory bodies. Their moral and legal duties ('moral' and 'ethical' can be treated as synonymous in normal discourse) are equally, if not more, significant. It is not *necessarily* the case that professional duties, as stated by professional regulatory bodies, are either legal or moral, although in most cases they will be. It might be argued that duties can be hierarchically ordered; if so, moral duties would be at the top of the hierarchy. Although exceptions are clearly possible, one would hope that the law is moral and that professional duties require practitioners to act both morally and legally.

What are the key moral duties relating to health-care research? It has already been argued that there is a moral duty to undertake research. It is not contentious to claim that patients have an entitlement to the best possible care and treatment, which necessarily entails research. If this were the sole duty of the health-care researcher, however, it would be legitimate to pursue any activity having this as its goal. In short, patients and healthy volunteers could be used or abused with impunity, as illustrated in the earlier examples. Proposed research can be analysed with reference to theories of ethics. Theories can be divided into those that relate to the motives of the moral agent and those that relate to acts.

Kantian ethical theory is possibly the best example of an agent-based, or deon-tological, theory (Eaton, 2004). The agent is required to adhere to strict duties, for example, not to lie. Kant starts from the question 'What ought I to do?' and searches for a supreme moral duty, which he calls the 'categorical imperative'. The categorical imperative, sometimes known as the 'golden rule', has been formulated in a variety of ways, the most common of which is: 'Act only on that maxim which at the same time you can will to be a universal law.' This maxim comes down to an obligation to 'do as you would be done by' and places the person at the heart of the theory. Kant reasons that, given that people are inclined to act morally and are therefore capable of moral activity, they are deserving of moral respect. For this reason, people should never be used as a means to an end; rather, they should be regarded as 'ends in themselves'.

The most superficial analysis of research activity reveals a need to use people as means to ends; this offends the fundamental basis of Kantian ethics. What of the research participant who freely volunteers to participate, as is often the case for patients with cancer when undergoing trials for new treatments? The Kantian position requires people to treat themselves with the same respect as they treat others; it is not acceptable to use oneself as a means to an end. Without further, increasingly complex argument, it can be concluded that no strong Kantian can readily approve of health-care research. It might also be concluded that any person of Kantian persuasion has morally defensible grounds for refusing to undertake or participate in human research.

Other moral theories relate to acts rather than the motives of the actor; the best known is utilitarianism (Goodin, 1995). Utilitarianism is an example of consequen-tialist ethics, where the focus is on the consequences of actions, in other words, ends. Foster (2001) argues that '[utilitarianism] has a place by right in our consid-eration of research, since research is about seeking and finding goals, or outcomes'. In determining the morality of an act, the agent is required to evaluate its outcome with regard to the degree to which it promotes human interests, with a proviso that every individual's interest should be treated equally. Various forms of utilitar-ianism identify different measures of 'interest' which include pleasure, happiness and, more recently, preferences and welfare (West, 2003). One of the main reasons for promoting human interests is human capacity to experience, for example, plea-sure and pain; in so far as other animals have this capacity, modern utilitarianism takes them into account. It is not always possible to promote positive outcomes, for example, the greatest pleasure. In this case an action may be ethical in so far as it promotes positive and/or minimizes negative outcomes. The moral defence of most health-care research lies in utilitarian reasoning. It may be acceptable to use a person, perhaps in a drugs trial, if the outcome is knowledge, which might be employed in achieving a greater good. But what if a greater good could be attained by abusing people, as in some of the examples of unethical research discussed earlier? This concern is sometimes advanced as a criticism of utilitarianism, along with further concerns about accuracy of prediction of outcomes and relative merits of different interests.

It is possible to employ utilitarianism when evaluating rules as well as acts. Although an act that promotes the welfare of a majority over the suffering of a minority might be considered moral, it is unlikely that many would agree that such a rule would be acceptable. Imagine a rule claiming that we *ought* to promote the welfare of the majority regardless of suffering caused to a minority. Such a rule is hardly calculated to promote overall human interests because we might all, with good reason, fear becoming part of that minority.

The ethical researcher, then, should be aiming to promote human interests and a proposed project will be ethical in so far as it is designed to do so. When considering the means to this end, most researchers will be confronted with a need to compromise some basic duties. The first priority is to establish whether it is absolutely necessary to compromise these duties. A great deal might be achieved by accessing a research population to whom no primary professional duty is owed. Health-care practitioners frequently research their 'own' patients and clients, producing an inevitable conflict of duty. When challenged, it becomes clear that often the reason for this is simply convenience.

The second priority is to minimize any potential harm or disadvantages that might arise. This could include provision of access to support organizations when respondents are interviewed on sensitive topics, for example 'living with cancer'. The administration of a placebo is a moral harm in so far as it is a deceit; it may also be a practical harm in that its consequence is deprivation of active treatment. Where harm, albeit minimal, is inevitable, the researcher is obliged to muster a robust moral defence. Where there is no known alternative to a trial drug and it is at least possible that it will have no positive effects beyond that of a placebo or, more contentiously, that potential harms in the form of side effects might outweigh any benefit, it may none the less be considered ethically justifiable to trial it, since the potential benefit could be great.

What are the legal duties of the researcher? Legal duties can be derived from statute law (acts of parliament) and case law. The most significant statute is the Human Rights Act 1998; all other law relating to health-care research should be read and interpreted in conjunction with this. In relation to health-care research, the most important provisions of the act include rights to life, liberty and privacy, and prohibition of discrimination. Some of the examples of unethical research discussed earlier violate the right to life. Research participants' rights to liberty and privacy must be protected by ensuring that they are aware of any infringements resulting from research, and that full consent is given. Law relating to consent is largely derived from case law and is considered later, from the perspective of the participant.

The issue of discrimination is interesting. A clear example of discrimination arises when researchers select participants using inclusion criteria other than those that are scientifically defensible or designed to protect vulnerable people, for example prisoners might be selected on the grounds that they are easy to monitor. It is equally possible to discriminate by exclusion. Participating in therapeutic research allows the possibility of gaining benefit; if a person were excluded on the grounds of, for example, not speaking English, this would be discriminatory. Therapeutic research entails testing a form of treatment on a person who might benefit. It should be emphasized that benefit is only a possibility and, for this reason, the distinction between therapeutic and non-therapeutic research is arguable; the primary intention of the researcher, in both cases, is acquisition of knowledge rather than provision of treatment.

Privacy can be considered in relation to the Data Protection Act 1998, which applies to all personal data identifying a participant. Researchers have a duty to gain consent from participants before accessing personal data, making it clear what the data will be used for. They are also obliged to anonymize any published data, ensuring participants' right to privacy. If researchers wish to access patient data held by a Trust, they must seek authorization from the data custodian, known as the Caldicott Guardian.

Having considered the duties of researchers in some detail, it is worth while considering whether they have any rights. The short answer is that they have the rights that are necessary to meet their duties, for example, a right to apply to an NHS research ethics committee (REC). Researchers do not have a right to undertake research; arguably they have duties to extend existing knowledge. However, researchers do have some legal rights, for example the right to a prompt response from an REC; this would normally be within 60 days (Medicines for Human Use (Clinical Trials) Regulations 2004).

THE RESEARCH

The objective of health-care research is acquisition of knowledge which enables provision of effective, evidence-based care and treatment. Conferring benefit on participants is rarely the immediate objective of the researcher, as discussed earlier; the likelihood is that the outcomes of the research will be used for the benefit of others. Perhaps the exception to this general principle is action research, where findings are continuously fed back into the field. In a typical randomized controlled clinical trial, participants enter a 'lottery' where they may or may not be allocated the trial drug, which may or may not be effective. Any benefit is largely a matter of chance. If, however, research proves a drug to be effective, there is normally an obligation to continue to provide it to all participants after the trial has concluded (World Medical Association, Declaration of Helsinki 2000).

It is not difficult to understand why all health-care research must be ethically reviewed. Given the comparatively recent examples of unethical research, it is not surprising that the DoH has produced governance arrangements for research in the NHS. These arrangements are known as 'Governance Arrangements for Research Ethics Committees' (GAfREC) (DoH, 2001b). The DoH requires all NHS research to be reviewed by an NHSREC. NHS research is defined in GAfREC as any research involving: patients, relatives and carers; staff access to data, organs and bodily material; and the use of NHS premises and facilities. It includes those who have recently died on NHS premises. The evolving plans to implement a national research ethics service (COREC, 2006) are likely to include some changes to the definition above. One issue under consideration is the withdrawal of the demand for ethical review of research involving only NHS staff as participants.

The primary purpose of RECs is to 'protect the dignity, safety and well-being of all actual or potential research participants' (DoH, 2001b). The RECs do have a secondary role with regard to researchers having consideration for their own interests and, more importantly, safety. Strictly speaking, RECs do not approve proposals, because researchers ultimately require the approval of appropriate managers and professionals in the specific locations in which the research takes place. RECs can provide a favourable opinion, a necessary requirement before commencement of any study. RECs are appointed by Strategic Health Authorities, but they are strictly independent and not in any way accountable to NHS Trusts. This ensures that proposals can be reviewed freely in the absence of any sort of coercion. The membership of RECs includes relevant health-care professionals, other experts, for example a scientific officer with knowledge of statistical analysis, and laity. Lay members are particularly important as they are more able to review a proposal from the participant's perspective. At least a third of the membership must comprise laity. There is an obligation for all members to undertake introductory and continuing training. It should be noted that membership of an REC is entirely voluntary.

On the implementation of the Medicines for Human Use (Clinical Trials) Regulations 2004, RECs were re-classified to take account of the requirement for a single ethical review. Any study receiving a favourable opinion from an REC is approved to take place in any location without further review. In this way, all RECs have become multicentre research ethics committees. However, RECs are designated as different types. Type 1 RECs only review phase 1 clinical trials involving healthy volunteers; type 2 and type 3 committees can review all other NHS research, including clinical trials of investigational medicinal products (CTIMPs); however, type 2 committees are restricted to CTIMPs on sites within their own Strategic Health Authorities. There are special committees to review genetic research and research involving prisoners.

A multicentre study can be designated as requiring site-specific assessment, which is undertaken by a subcommittee of the local REC. This does not conduct a further review; its task is limited to evaluating the proposal with regard to locality issues, including consideration of resources and availability of a local, suitably qualified researcher. An application to an REC should be viewed as one of the last stages before commencement of a project. RECs expect complete documentation providing evidence that the project has been peer reviewed or, in the case of a small-scale student project, that it is appropriately supervised. Where necessary, applications should also provide evidence that the proposal has received the support of the relevant Trust's research and development department, that is, that it has management approval. It is equally important to provide evidence of compliance with the provisions of the Data Protection Act 1998. In summary, in order to gain the favourable opinion of an REC, proposed research must meet the conditions stated above and:

- comply with the Declaration of Helsinki
- comply with European and national law
- demonstrate that the researcher has met their moral, legal and professional duties
- meet the criteria stated in sections 9.13−9.18 of GAfREC (DoH, 2001b).

THE PARTICIPANT

It should now be clear that participating in research is likely to be, at least in part, an act of altruism. Direct benefit to research participants is unlikely to be a primary endpoint of many research projects, although there are, of course, exceptions. Normally, any benefits accrued will be a matter of chance and most participants will find themselves suffering some disadvantage in the interests of health-care advancement. The welfare of all participants is obviously important but it should be noted that there is a real danger that some people who are suffering from the most serious conditions, including some cancers, will see themselves as having little to lose. These people, along with other vulnerable individuals, including minors and people experiencing mental disorders, are particularly in need of protection.

When considering the welfare of participants, an obvious starting point is to enquire whether or not the research is necessary and worth while. The DoH (2001c) states:

It is essential that existing sources of evidence, especially systematic reviews, are considered carefully prior to undertaking research. Research which duplicates other work unnecessarily or which is not of sufficient quality to contribute something useful to existing knowledge is in itself unethical.

This stance undoubtedly jeopardizes many student projects that aim to employ primary data collection; however, it is difficult to argue that the interests of participants can reasonably be subordinated to the interests of students. Research based on secondary data, or simply designing a potential project, will meet most reasonable learning outcomes. It should be noted, however, that most RECs are sympathetic to students' learning needs and do not rigidly apply the restriction quoted above. The proposed research still has to meet general ethical requirements but its quality need not be questioned if it only involves minimal inconvenience to participants and they are fully informed of the status of the study.

Worthwhile research should, wherever possible, be designed to minimize risks and disadvantages to participants. A good example of such a strategy is the decision to use a control arm only when it is absolutely necessary. Participants acting as controls usually receive placebo 'treatment' or no treatment at all. Although they avoid risks associated with the trial treatment, they may suffer as a result of being deprived of an alternative, active treatment.

Research that has been well designed can still pose risks to participants. A recent phase 1 trial (where drugs are tested on healthy volunteers for the first time) gained much publicity when six men suffered serious reactions to the trial drug, TGN1412. Headlines such as 'Elephant man given drug too quickly' (Deer, 2006) captured the severity of the near-fatal reaction. Interestingly, the trial drug was being developed to treat, amongst other conditions, leukaemia. The Secretary of State for Health established an Expert Scientific Group (ESG) to investigate matters surrounding this trial (DoH, 2006). In the ESG's final recommendations there was a suggestion that, in trials of drugs with known cellular toxicity, it might be appropriate for patients with cancer to participate, rather than healthy volunteers. This was on the grounds that there was at least some potential for benefit, though the authors made the strong point that the overriding concern should always be the 'rights, safety, and well-being of volunteers whether patients or healthy individuals' (DoH, 2006).

It is essential to ensure that all participants are made fully aware of the implications of their participation. They should be given clear information and sufficient time to reflect upon it, as well as opportunities to discuss it with others. Consent is an absolute requirement, and that consent should be real. To meet UK legal obligations, it must be freely given, in the absence of any sort of inducement or coercion and in the light of sufficient information, and the participant must have the mental capacity to understand the implications of their participation. The Mental Capacity Act 2005 permits, in some circumstances, research involving incapacitated adults; this is discussed further later. All participants must be assured that their (continuing) participation is entirely voluntary and without prejudice to any normal care and treatment that they might otherwise receive.

Well-designed research may still entail the collection of sensitive data and other material, including tissue, which may have serious implications for the participant. The nature of data collected must be made explicit to the participant, whose privacy must be safeguarded as far as possible; this can be achieved by collecting the minimum data necessary and treating it in confidence. Participant confidentiality is protected by the legal and professional duties discussed earlier.

The ethical considerations of participants can be identified in relation to key stages of the research process, including:

- identifying potential participants
- recruiting participants
- informing participants
- gaining participants' consent.

Research participants are typically identified using inclusion and exclusion criteria determined by the scientific design of the study. There are, however, overriding ethical concerns. Unless they are necessary participants of a particular study, it is normal to exclude vulnerable people. Vulnerable people include those who are seriously ill, those whose freedoms are compromised and those lacking capacity. It is normal to exclude terminally ill people, prisoners, minors, people with serious mental disorders and any other person who does not have the capacity to understand the nature and implications of their involvement, that is, any person who cannot realistically consent to participation. Some research does involve vulnerable people; how could effective care and treatment for this group be provided without some research directly involving them? With regard to mentally incapacitated adults, the Mental Capacity Act 2005 makes some provision for research. This provision is limited to research connected to the condition which has brought about their incapacity and, furthermore, it must be ascertained that research of comparable quality could not have been undertaken with people with the capacity to consent. A carer (not a paid carer) must legally be consulted regarding the participation of a mentally incapacitated adult in research. If the carer's view is that the person would not wish to take part in the particular project then that decision is binding. It is the role of the NHSREC to determine whether proposed research satisfies the aforementioned legal requirements; thus a favourable opinion from an REC is a legal and ethical requirement before research involving incapacitated adults can be undertaken.

A person holding parental responsibility for a minor can consent on his or her behalf; given the provisions of the Children Act 1989, they should assure themselves that the welfare interests of the minor are not jeopardized.

Participants should be invited to join a study, that is, they should be given the opportunity to opt in. It is unethical to require participants to opt out. This basic requirement is easily breached. An example might be sending a postal questionnaire to a potential participant and requiring them to inform the researcher if they do not wish to participate. Furthermore, imagine the potential distress arising from receiving a questionnaire including sensitive topics, without any prior warning. In most cases it is normal to send a letter of invitation, with an accompanying information sheet, seeking the participant's agreement to join a study. Potential participants may, of course, be approached directly or through a third party; in any event, comprehensible information, ideally in writing, is an absolute requirement.

When a questionnaire is directly administered, information may be given orally or may comprise an introductory paragraph on the questionnaire itself. The National Research Ethics Service provides templates for information sheets and consent forms. These can be easily accessed via the office's web site at www.nres.npsa.nhs.uk. It should be noted that information sheets and consent forms must be on headed paper, include dates and version numbers, and provide the researcher's contact details. The reason information is so important is that real consent is dependent on it. Consent, again, is an absolute requirement. Consent need not necessarily be in writing; for example, completion and return of a simple questionnaire by an informed participant may reasonably be taken as evidence of consent. But in most cases, written consent will be necessary. It is normally taken at the time of participation by the researcher, who must ensure that the participant has had sufficient time to consider the implications of involvement. A consent form must include evidence of the participant's general willingness to join the study based on information received, their right to withdraw without negative consequences and explicit consent where sensitive data are collected. Examples of the last include photographs, video and audio recordings, data from medical records and data derived from tissue and other specimens. Participants must be informed of the overall management of the data, for example, audio recordings are normally transcribed and the original tape either destroyed or erased. Any data or other material retained for future use must be brought to the attention of the participant. The most contentious example in this category is retained tissue.

Retained tissue is particularly significant in research on cancer care and treatment. Tumour cells are frequently collected in the course of therapeutic and non-therapeutic research; in the former, research might be conducted on the cells to find the most effective chemotherapeutic regimen, thus directly benefiting the patient. In the latter, retained cells might be used in the course of developing drugs that would benefit others. Given concerns raised by the unethical retention of organs and tissue, the Human Tissue Act 2004 included measures legally regulating the use of tissue for research purposes. Briefly, tissue can only be retained for research purposes with the explicit consent of the patient. Alternatively, a researcher can legally use anonymized samples of tissue as long as they have the consent of an appropriate REC (Brazier, 2006).

Although tissue is normally anonymized, there are typically coded links such that, in the event of significant information coming to light, it is possible to contact the donor. The importance of research involving tissue donated by cancer patients cannot be overstated. It is worth noting that the unethical retention of organs and tissue in the past could negatively impact on this research now, because potential donors or their relatives may have serious concerns. This is perhaps one of the most compelling grounds for ensuring that research is always ethical.

One final ethical issue remains. At the beginning of this chapter, it was argued that research is ethically sensitive because it frequently entails the use of people for the benefit of others. No benefit can be gained unless the results of research are successfully disseminated. On this ground, publication of research is a moral duty. In other words, the endpoint of valuable research should never be simply the award of a degree or promotion of personal or institutional status.

Glossary

Allele	One of several alternative forms of a gene occupying the same locus on a chromosome.
Angiogenesis	Formation of new blood vessels.
Apoptosis	Programmed cell death.
ATP	Adenosine triphosphate.
Cancer	Uncontrolled proliferation and growth of cells into other tissues.
CDK	Cyclin-dependent kinases.
Cell	Basic unit of all living matter.
Cellular senescence	Limited capacity of cells to divide beyond a finite number of population doublings.
CFCs	Chlorofluorocarbons.
Chromatin	DNA$-$protein complex containing genes in the cell.
Codon	Three adjacent nucleotides in a nucleic acid that code for one amino acid.
Deoxyribose	The five-carbon sugar with hydrogen at the $2'$ position found in DNA. Different from the ribose sugar found in RNA.
Diploid	A cell containing two sets of chromosomes $-$ the number found in normal somatic cells.
DNA	Deoxyribonucleic acid.
DNA ligase	An enzyme that seals together two DNA fragments.
DNA polymerase	An enzyme that links complementary nucleotides together to replicate DNA.
Endoplasmic reticulum	Series of inter-connecting tubular tunnels in the cell.
Epigenetic	Non-genetic changes that alter an organism's phenotype, such as methylation.
Eukaryotic	An animal or plant that has a membrane-bound nucleus and organelles.
Exon	A segment of DNA that is expressed by a mature RNA product.
Germ cell	Precursor cells that give rise to sperm or eggs.
Germline	The lineage of germ cells.

The Biology of Cancer, Second Edition. Edited by J. Gabriel
© 2007 John Wiley & Sons, Ltd.

Golgi apparatus	A structure that modifies proteins and fats in the cell.
HAMAs	Human anti-mouse monoclonal antibodies.
Haploid	Cells containing only one set of chromosomes – usually germ cells.
Hydrogen Bond	A chemical bond in which a hydrogen atom of one molecule is attracted to a negatively charged atom, especially a nitrogen, oxygen or fluorine atom, usually of another molecule.
IHC	Immunohistochemistry.
Introns	Non-coding DNA sequences separating the coding exons. During gene expression these introns are removed from the mature RNA by splicing.
Locus	Site of a gene on a chromosome.
LREC	Local research ethics committee.
Lysosomes	Spherical bodies in the cell, containing digestive enzymes.
mAb	Monoclonal antibody.
Metastasis	Spread of a primary cancer to another part of the body.
Mitochondria	Bodies in the cell that break down sugar molecules in the presence of oxygen and produce energy in the form of ATP.
Mitosis	Cell division.
MMPs	Matrix metalloproteins.
Monogenic	Controlled by, or associated with, a single gene.
Monomer	A single molecule that has the ability to combine with identical or similar molecules to form a polymer.
MREC	Multicentre research ethics committee.
Nuclear envelope	Double-layered membrane protecting and separating the nucleus from the cytoplasm and molecules in the cell.
Nucleolus	Part of the cell nucleus which produces ribosomes.
Nucleosome	A structural unit of chromatin.
Nucleotide	The basic sub-units of nucleic acids, which are made up of a pyrimidine or purine base, a pentose sugar and a phosphate group.
Organelles	Subcellular functional components of a cell, e.g. the nucleus.
PCR	Polymerase chain reaction.
Pentose	A sugar containing five carbon molecules.
Polygenic	Controlled by, or associated with, more than one gene.
Promoter	A site on DNA that is upstream ($5'$) of the coding sequence, to which RNA polymerase enzymes bind, and which initiates their transcription.
PSA	Prostate-specific antigen.

Ribose	A pentose sugar found in the nucleotides of RNA.
Ribosomes	Organelles made of rRNA and protein. These are the protein-making machinery.
RNA	Ribonucleic acid.
Somatic cell	All cells of an organism except those of the germline.

References

Abbass, A.K. and Lichtman, A.H. (2006) *Basic Immunology: Functions and Disorders of the Immune System*, 2nd edn, Elsevier, Philadelphia.

Abbott, A. (2006) Cancer: The root of the problem. *Nature*, **442**, 742–3.

Abgrall, S., Orbach, D., Bonhomme-Faivre, L. and Orbach-Arbous S. (2002) Tumours in organ transplant recipients may give clues to their control by immunity. *Anticancer Research* **22**, 3597–604.

Abutalib, S.A. and Tallman, M.S. (2006) Monoclonal antibodies for the treatment of acute myeloid leukemia. *Current Pharmaceutical Biotechnology*, **7**, 343–69.

Adams, J., Carder, P.J., Downey, S. *et al.* (2000) Vascular Endothelial Growth Factor (VEGF) in breast cancer: Comparison of plasma, serum, and tissue VEGF and microvessel density and effects of tamoxifen1. *Cancer Research*, **60**, 2898–905.

Alberts, B., Johnson, A., Lewis, J. *et al.* (2002) Internal organisation of the cell. In: *Molecular Biology of the Cell*, 4th edn, Garland Publishing, New York and London.

Allen, G.E. (2003) Mendel and modern genetics: The legacy for today. *Endeavour*, **27**, 63–8.

Allen, R.E. [1990] *The Concise Oxford Dictionary of Current English*, 8th edn, Clarenden Press, Oxford.

Allwood, M., Stanley, A. and Wright, A.P. (eds) (2002) *The Cytotoxics Handbook*, 4th edn, Radcliffe Medical Press, Oxford.

Altfeld, M. and Rosenberg, E.S. (2000) The role of CD4+ T helper cells in the cytotoxic T lymphocyte response to HIV. *Curr Opin Immunel* **12**, 375–80.

American Society of Clinical Oncology (ASCO) (1996) Clinical practice guidelines for the use of tumor markers in breast and colorectal cancer. *Journal Clinical Oncology*, **14**, 2843–77.

American Society of Clinical Oncology (ASCO) (1998) 1997 update and recommendations for the use of tumor markers in breast and colorectal cancer. *Journal Clinical Oncology*, **16**, 793–5.

American Society of Clinical Oncology (ASCO) (1999) 1998 update of recommended breast cancer surveillance guideline. *Journal Clinical Oncology*, **16**, 793–5.

American Urological Association (AUA) (2000) Prostate-specific antigen (PSA) best practice policy. *Oncology*, **14**, 267–72, 277–8, 280 passim. http://www.cancernetwork.com/journals/oncology (Accessed Nov 2002).

Andre, F.T. (2003) Vaccinology: Past achievements, present roadblocks and future promises. *Vaccine*, **21**, 593–5.

Andreeff, M., Goodrich, D.W. and Pardee, A.B. (2000) Cell proliferation, differentiation, and apoptosis. In: *Cancer Medicine*, 5th edn (eds R.C. Bast, Jr, D.W. Kufe, R.E. Pollock, R.R. Weichselbaum, J.F. Holland, E. Frei, III and T.S. Gansler), BC Decker Inc, Canada.

Anonymous. (1996) Clinical practice guidelines for the use of tumor markers in breast and colorectal cancer. Adopted on 17 May 1996 by American Society of Clinical Oncology. *J. Clin. Oncol.*, **14**, 2843−77.

Anonymous. (2001) Porton Down Probe launched. *The Guardian*, 30 July 2001.

Anonymous. (2006) *British National Formulary*, 52nd edn, BMJ Publishing Group & The Pharmaceutical Press, London.

Antequera, F., Boyes, J. and Bird, A. (1990) High levels of de novo methylation and altered chromatin structure at CpG islands in cell lines. *Cell*, **62**, 503−14.

Apoptosis Information (2007) Retrieved 11 Feb 2007 from http://en.wikipedia.org/wiki/apoptosis.

Appay,V. and Rowland-Jones, S.L. (2002) Premature aging of the immune system: The cause of AIDS. *Trends in Immunology*, **23**(12), 580−5.

Ardeshna, K.M., Smith, P., Norton, A. *et al.* (2003) Long term effect of a watch and wait policy versus immediate systemic treatment for asymptomatic advanced stage non-Hodgkins Lymphoma: A randomised controlled trial. *Lancet*, **362**(9383), 516−22.

Armstrong, A.C. and Hawkins, R.E. (2001) Vaccines in oncology: Background and clinical potential. *Vaccines*, **74**, 991−1002.

Armstrong, K., Eisen, A. and Weber, B. (2000) Assessing the risk of breast cancer. *New Engl J Med*, **342**(8), 564−71.

Arteaga, C.L. (2001) The epidermal growth factor receptor: from mutant oncogene in nonhuman cancers to therapeutic target in human neoplasia. *J. Clin. Oncol*, **19**, 32S−40S.

Association of Clinical Biochemists in Ireland (1999) Guidelines for the use of tumor markers, http://www.iol.ie/deskenny/acbi.html (Accessed Oct 2002).

Avery, O.T., Macleod, C.M. and McCarty, M. (1944) Studies on the chemical nature of the substance introducing transformation of pneumococcal types. *J. Exp. Med*, **79**, 137−58.

Bailar, J.C. and Gornik, H.L. (1997) Cancer undefeated. *N Engl J Med*, **336**, 1569−74.

Baildam, A., Keeling, F., Noble, M. *et al.* (2001) Nurse led follow-up for women treated for breast cancer: A randomized controlled trial. *European Journal of Surgical Oncology*, **27**(8), 792.

Baker, C., Wuest, J. and Norager-Stern, P. (1992) Method slurring: The grounded theory/phenomenology example. *Journal of Advanced Nursing*, **17**, 1355−60.

Balmain, A. (2001) Cancer genetics: From Boveri and Mendel to microarrays. *Nat Rev Cancer*, **1** (1), 77−82.

Balmain A., Gray, J. and Ponder, B. (2003) The genetics and genomics of cancer. *Nat Genet*, **33** Suppl: 238−44.

Baselga, J. and Albanell, J. (2001) Mechanism of action of anti-HER-2 monoclonal antibodies. *Annals of Oncology*, **12**(Suppl 1), S35−S41.

Baselga, J., Norton, L., Albanell, J., Kim, Y.M. and Mendelsohn, J. (1998) Recombinant humanized anti-HER-2 antibody (Herceptin) enhances the anti-tumour activity of paclitaxel and doxorubicin against HER-2/neu overexpressing human breast cancer xenografts. *Cancer Research*, **58**, 2825−31.

Bast, R.C., Ravdin, P., Hayes, D.F. *et al.* (2001) 2000 update of recommendations for the use of tumor markers in breast and colorectal cancer: Clinical practice guidelines of the American Society of Clinical Oncology [Erratum]. *J Clin Oncol*, **19**, 4185−88.

Baylin, S.B. and Herman, J.G. (2000) DNA hypermethylation in tumourigenesis. *TIG*, **16**(4), 168−74.

Baylin, S.B., Belinsky, S.A. and Herman, J.G. (2000) Aberrant methylation of gene promoters in cancer — concepts, misconcepts, and promise. *J. Natl. Cancer Inst*, **92**, 1460–61.

Becknell, B. and Caligiuri, M.A. (2003) Cancer T-cell therapy expands. *Nature Medicine*, **9**, 257–58.

Bell, R. (2002) Duration of therapy in metastatic breast cancer: Management using Herceptin. *Anticancer Drugs*, **12**, 561–8.

Bellmut, J., Ribas, A., Eres, N. *et al.* (1997) Carboplatin based versus cisplatin based chemotherapy in the treatment of surgically incurable advanced bladder carcinoma. *Cancer*, **80**(10), 1966–72.

Berd, D. (1998) Cancer vaccines: Reborn or just recycled. *Seminars in Oncology*, **25**, 605–10.

Berd, D. (2001) Autologous, hapten-modified vaccine as treatment for human cancers. *Vaccine*, **19**, 2565–70.

Berger, M.S., Leopold, L.H., Dowell, J.A., Korth-Bradley, J.M. and Sherman, M.L. (2002) Licensure of gemtuzumab ozogamicin for the treatment of selected patients 60 years of age and older with acute myeloid leukemia in first relapse. *Investigational New Drugs*, **20**, 395–406.

Berry, D., Dakhit, S., Modiano, M. *et al.* (2002) Phase III study of mitoxantrone plus low dose prednisolone versus low dose prednisolone alone in patients with asymptomatic hormone refractory prostate cancer. *J Urol*, **168**(6), 2451–53.

Bidart, J.M., Thuillier, F., Augereau, C. *et al.* (1999) Kinetics of serum tumor marker concentrations and usefulness in clinical monitoring. *Clinical Chemistry*, **45**(10), 1690–707.

Bird, A. (1992) The essentials of DNA methylation. *Cell*, **70**, 5–8.

Birmingham, K. (2002) What is translational oncology. *Nature Medicine*, **8**, 647.

Black, N. (1994) Why do we need qualitative research. *Journal of Epidemilogy and Community Health*, **48**, 425–26.

Blackledge, G. and Averbuch, S. (2004) Gefitinib ('Iressa', ZD1839) and new epidermal growth factor receptor inhibitors. *Br J Cancer*, **90**, 566–72.

Blagosklomy, M. (2002) From the war on cancer to translational oncology. *Cancer Biology and Therapy*, July.

Bodey B, Body, B., Jr, Siegel, S. and Kiaser H.E. (2000) Failure of cancer vaccines: the significant limitations of this approach to immunotherapy. *Anticancer Research*, **20**, 2665–76.

Bonfrer, J.M.G., Duffy, M.J., Radtke, M. *et al.* (1999) Tumor markers in gynaecological cancers: EGTM recommendations. *Anticancer Res*, **19**, 2807–10.

Bonnadonna, G., Brusamoline, E., Valagussa, P. *et al.* (1976) Combination chemotherapy as an adjuvant treatment in operable breast cancer. *N Engl J Med*, **294**, 405–10.

Bonnet, D. and Dick, J.E. (1997) Human acute myeloid leukemia is organized as a hierarchy that originates from a primitive hematopoietic cell. *Nat. Med*, **3**, 730–7.

Boon, T. and Van den Enbde, B. (2003) Tumour immunology. *Current Opinions in Immunology*, **15**, 129–30.

Booy, E.P., Johar, D., Maddika, S. *et al.* (2006) Monoclonal and bispecific antibodies as novel therapeutics. *Arch Immunol Ther Exp (Warsz)*, **54**(2), 85–101.

Bowling, A. (1997) *Research Methods in Health: Investigating Health and Health Services*, Open University Press, Buckingham.

Bowling, A. (2001) *Measuring Disease*, 2nd edn, Open University Press, Buckingham.

Brazier, M., Forargue, S. A brief guide to the Human Tissue Act 2004. *Clinical Ethics*, Volume 1, Number 1, March 2006, pp. 26–32 (7).

Breaden, K. (1997) Cancer and beyond: The question of survivorship. *Journal of Advanced Nursing*, **26**, 978–84.

Breivik, J. and Gaudernack, G. (1999) Genomic instability, DNA methylation, and natural selection in colorectal carcinogenesis. *Semin Cancer Biol*, **9**, 245–54.

Bremers, A.T.J., Kuppen, P.J.K. and Parmiani, G. (2000) Tumour immunotherapy: The adjuvant treatment of the 21st century. *European Journal of Surgical Oncology*, **26**, 418–24.

Brennan, P. and Croft, P. (1994) Interpreting the results of observational research: Chance in not such a fine thing. *BMJ*, **309**, 727–30.

British Medical Association (BMA) (1997) *Family Health Encyclopaedia*, BMA Books, London.

Bromberg, J.E., Siemers, M.D. and Taphoorn, M.J. (2002) Is a "vanishing tumour" always a lymphoma? *Neurology*, **59**(5), 762–4.

Buchsel, P.C. and DeMeyer, E.S. (2006) Dendritic cells. Emerging roles in tumour immunotherapy. *Clinical Journal of Oncology Nursing*, **10**(5), 629–40.

Buckley, R.H. (2003) Transplantation immunology: Organ and bone marrow. *J Allergy Clinical Immunology*, **112**(2 Suppl), S733–S744.

Burnet, F.M. (1967) Immunological aspects of malignant disease. *Lancet*, **1**, 1171–74.

Burns, E.A. (2004) Effects of aging on immune system. *The Journal of Nutrition, Health and Aging*, **8**(1), 9–18.

Burns, E.A. and Leventhal, E.A. (2000) Aging, immunity and cancer. *Cancer Control*, **7**, 513–22.

Burton, C., Linch, D., Hoskin, P. *et al.* (2006) A phase III trial comparing CHOP to PMitCEBO with or without G-CSF in patients aged sixty plus with aggressive non-Hodgkins lymphoma. *Br J Cancer*, **94**(6), 806–13.

Bustin, S.A. (2005) Real-time, fluorescence-based quantitative PCR: A snapshot of current procedures and preferences. *Expert Rev Mol Diagn*, **5**, 493–8.

Cahill, D.P., Lengauer, C., Yu, J. *et al.* (1998) Mutations of mitotic checkpoint genes in human cancers. *Nature*, **392**, 300–3.

Cairncross, G., Berkley, B., Shaw, E. *et al.* (2006) Phase III trial of chemotherapy plus radiotherapy compared with radiotherapy alone for pure and mixed anaplastic oligodendroglioma: Intergroup Radiation Therapy Oncology Group Trial 9402. *J Clin Oncol*, **24**(18), 2707–14.

Cancer Research UK:

Specific Cancers Colorectoral (bowel) cancer (2002) www.cancerhelp.org.uk/help/default.asp? Page=2806 (accessed 11.02.07)

Specific Cancers Breast cancer (2002) www.cancerhelp.org.uk/help/default.asp? Page=3284 (accessed 11.02.07)

Specific Cancers Lung cancer (2002) www.cancerhelp.org.uk/help/default.asp? Page=2964 (accessed 11.02.07)

Specific Cancers Melanoma skin cancer (2002) www.cancerhelp.org.uk/help/default.asp? Page=3009 (accessed 11.02.07)

CancerVOICES (2002) News, views and action. *Cancervoices*, **7, 4.**

Cao, Y. and Lam, L. (2003) Bispecific antibody conjugate in therapeutics. *Advanced Drug Delivery Reviews*, **55**, 171–9.

Carter, P., Presta, L., Gorman, C.M. *et al.* (1992) Humanization of an anti-p185HER-2 antibody for human cancer therapy. *Proceedings of the National Academy of Sciences of the USA*, **89**, 4285–9.

Cartmel, B., Reid, M. (2000) Cancer control and epidemiology. In: Greonwald, S., Frogge, M., Goodman, M. and Yarbo, C. (eds), *Cancer Nursing: Principles and Practice*, 5 edn, Jones and Bartlett, Boston, MA.

Cell Cycle Animation (2006) Retrieved 11 Feb 2007 from http://www.cellsalive.com/toc_cellbio.htm.

Cella, D., Tulsky, D., Gray, G. *et al.* (1993) The functional assessment of cancer therapy scale: Development and validation of the general measure. *Journal of Clinical Oncology*, **11**(3), 570–9.

Central Office of Research Ethics Committees (2006) *Building on Improvement: Implementing the Recommendations of the Ad Hoc Advisory Group on the Operation of NHS Research Ethics Committees*, National Patient Safety Agency, London.

Chambers, A.F. and Matrisian, L.M. (1997) Changing views of the role of matrix metalloproteinases in metastasis. *J. Natl. Cancer Inst*, **89**, 1260–70.

Chang, S.M., Theodosopoulos, P., Lamborn, K. *et al.* (2004) Temozolamide in the treatment of recurrent malignant glioma. *Cancer*, **100**(3), 605–11.

Chargaff, E., Lipshitz, R., Green, C. and Hodes, M.E. (1951) The composition of the deoxyribonucleic acid of salmon sperm. *J. Biol. Chem*, **192**, 223–30.

Chen, J., Flurkey, K. and Harrison, D.E. (2002) A reduced peripheral blood CD4+ lymphocyte proportion is a consistent ageing phenotype. *Mechanisms Ageing and Development*, **13**, 1445–53.

Cheson, B.D. (2001) Some like it hot. *Journal of Clinical Oncology*, **19**, 3908–11.

Cheson, B.D. (2003) Radioimmunotherapy of non-Hodgkins lymphoma. *Blood*, **101**(2), 391–8.

Chester, J.D., Dent, J.T., Wilson, G. *et al.* (2000) Protracted infusional 5-fluorouracil (5-FU) with bolus mitomycin in 5-FU resistant colorectal cancer. *Ann Oncol*, **11**(2), 235–7.

Cheung, K.L., Rosamund, C., Graves, L. and Robertson, J.F.R. (2002) Autoantibodies as circulating cancer markers. In: *Tumor Markers: Physiology, Pathobiology, Technology and Clinical Applications* (eds E.P. Diamandis, H. Fritsche, M.K. Schwartz and D.W. Chan), AACC Press, Chicago, pp. 123–32.

Ciberra, M.T., Rosinol, L., Ramiro, L. *et al.* (2006) Long term results of thalidomide in refractory and relapsed multiple myeloma with emphasis on response duration. *Eur J Haematol*, **77**(6), 486–92.

Clarke, M.F. (2004) Neurobiology at the root of brain cancer. *Nature*, **432**, 281–2.

Coghlan, A. (1991) The second chance for antibodies. *New Scientist*, **19**, 34–9.

Cohen, M. (1987) A historical overview of the phenomenological movement. *Image: Journals of Nursing Scholarship*, **19**(1), 31–4.

Colaizzi, P.F. (1978) Psychological research as the phenomenologist views it. In: *Existential Phenomenological Alternatives for Psychology* (eds R. Valle and M. King), Oxford University Press, Oxford, pp. 48–71.

Collins, A.T., Berry, P.A., Hyde, C., Stower, M.J. and Maitlandm, N.J. (2005) Prospective identification of tumorigenic prostate cancer stem cells. *Cancer Res*, **65**, 10946–51.

Collins, F.S., Patrinos, A., Jordan, E., Chakravarti, A., Gesteland, R., Walters, L. (1998) New goals for the US Human Genome Project: 1998–2003. *Science*, **23**, 682–9.

Cook, T., Reeves, J., Lanigan, A. and Stanton, P. (2001) Her-2 as prognostic and predictive marker for breast cancer. *Annals of Oncology*, **12**(Suppl 1), S23–S28.

Cope, D. (1995) Functions of a breast cancer support group as perceived by the participants: An ethnographic study. *Cancer Nursing*, **18**(6), 472–8.

Corner, J. (2001) What is cancer? In: *Cancer Nursing Care in Context* (eds J. Corner and C. Bailey), Blackwell Publishing, Oxford.

Corner J. (2002) Nurses' experiences of cancer. *European Journal of Cancer Care*, **11**, 193—9.

Corner, J. and Bailey, C. (eds) (2001) *Cancer Nursing Care in Context*, Blackwell Publishing, Oxford.

Cornwell, J. (1997) Cancer: The war against it. *Sunday Times*, 1 June, 14—9.

Coskun, U., Gunel, N., Onuk, E. *et al.* (2003) Effect of different neoadjuvant chemotherapy regimens on locally advanced breast cancer. *Neoplasma*, **50**(3), 210—16.

Costello, R.T., Fauriat, C., Gastaut, J.-A. and Olive, D. (2003) New approaches in the immunotherapy of haematological malignancies. *European J Haematology*, **70**, 333—45.

Cox, K. (1998) Investigating psychosocial aspects of participation in early anti-cancer drug trials: towards a choice of methodology. *Journal of Advanced Nursing*, **27**, 488—96.

Cox, K. (1999) Researching research: Patients' experiences of participation in phase 1 and II anti-cancer drug trials. *European Journal of Oncology Nursing*, **3**, 143—52.

Crawford, J. (2002) Pegfilgrastim administered once per cycle reduces incidence of chemotherapy-induced neutropenia (Review). *Drug*, **62**(Suppl 1), 89—98.

Crist, J. and Tanner, C. (2003) Interpretation/analysis methods in hermenutic interpretive phenomenology. *Nursing Research*, **52**(3), 202—5.

Culy, C. (2005) Bevacizumab: Antiangiogenesis cancer therapy. *Drugs Today*, **41**, 23—6.

Cunningham, D. (1995) Chemotherapy for solid tumours; an important progress in treatment. *BMJ*, **310**, 247—8.

Cutliffe, J. (2000) Methodological issues in grounded theory. *Journal of Advanced Nursing*, **31**(6), 1470—84.

Danenberg, P.V., Malli, H. and Swenson, S. (1999) Thymidylate synthase inhibitors. *Semin Oncol*, **26**(6), 621—31.

Davidson, E.J., Kitchener, H.C. and Stern, P.L. (2002) The use of vaccines in the prevention and treatment of cervical cancer. *Clinical Oncology*, **14**, 193—200.

Davies, C.G., Gallo, M.L. and Corvalan, R.F. (1999) Transgenic mice as a source of fully human antibodies for the treatment of cancer. *Cancer and Metastasis Review*, **18**, 421—5.

Davies, H., Bignell, G.R., Cox, C. *et al.* (2002) Mutations of the BRAF gene in human cancer. *Nature*, **417**, 949—54.

Dearden, C. (2002) Monoclonal antibody therapy of haematological malignancies (Therapy review). *Biodrugs*, **16**, 283—301.

Deer, B. (2006) Elephant Man given drug 'too quickly', *Sunday Times*, 24th September.

DeNardo, G.L., Sysko, V.V. and DeNardo, S.J. (2006) Cure of incurable lymphoma. *International Journal Radiation Oncology Biology Physics*, **66**, S46—S56.

De Witt, R., Roberts, J.T., Wilkinson, P.M. *et al.* (2001) Equivalence of 3 cycle BEP versus 4 cycles and of the 5 day schedule versus 3 days per cycle in good-prognosis germ cell cancer: A randomised study of the European Organisation for Research and Treatment of Cancer Genitourinary Tract Cancer Cooperative Group and the Medical Research Council. *J Clin Oncol*, **19**, 1629—40.

Dillman, R.O. (1989) Monoclonal antibodies for treating cancer. *Annals of Internal Medicine*, **111**, 592—603.

Dillman, R.O. (2002) Radiolabeled anti-CD20 monoclonal antibodies for the treatment of B-cell lymphoma. *Journal of Clinical Oncology*, **20**, 3545—57.

DOH (1995) *Calman—Hine Report. Framework for Commissioning Cancer Services*, DoH, London.

DOH (1999) The Royal Liverpool Children's Inquery Report. The Stationery Office, London.

DoH (2000a) *The NHS Cancer Plan*, DoH, London.

DoH (2000b) *Manual of Cancer Standards*, DoH, London.

DoH (2000c) *Towards a Strategy for Nursing Research and Development: Proposals for Action*, DoH, London.

DoH (2000d) *The Nursing Contribution to Cancer Care*, DoH, London.

DoH (2000e) *Report of a Census of Organs and Tissues Retained by Pathology Services in England*, The Stationery Office, London.

DoH (2000f) CEM/CMO/2000/15.

DoH (2001a) *The NHS Cancer Plan: Making Progress*, DoH, London.

DoH (2001b) *Governance Arrangements for Research Ethics Committees*, The Stationery Office, London.

DoH (2002) *National Patient Survey*, DoH, London.

DoH (2003a) *The Use of Human Organs and Tissue — An Interim Statement*, DoH, London.

DoH (2003b) *The Isaacs Report*, The Stationery Office, London.

DoH (2003c) *The Medicines for Human Use (Clinical Trials) Regulations*, DoH, London.

DoH (2004) *The Manual for Cancer Services*, DoH, London.

DoH (2005) *Referral Guidelines for Suspected Cancer*, DoH, London.

DoH (2006) *Best Research for Best Health*, DoH, London.

Downward, J., Yarden, Y., Mayes, E. *et al.* (1984) Close similarity of epidermal growth factor receptor and v-erb-B oncogene protein sequences. *Nature*, **307**, 521−7.

Draper, G., Little, M., Sorahan, T. *et al.* (1997) Cancer in the offspring of radiation workers: A record linkage study. *BMJ*, **315**, 1181−88.

Duffy, M.J. and McGing, P. (2005) *Association of Clinical Biochemists in Ireland*, 3rd edn, Guidelines for the use of tumor markers, http://www.acbi.ie/tm%20booklet%203rd%20edition%202005.pdf (Accessed Nov 2006).

Duffy, M.J., VanDalen, A. and Haglund, C. (2003) Clinical utility of biochemical markers in colorectal cancer: European Group on Tumor Markers (EGTM) guidelines. *Eur J Cancer*, **39**, 718−27.

Dumontet, C. and Sikic, B.I. (1999) Mechanisms of action of and resistance to anti-tubulin agents: Microtubule dynamics, drug transport and cell death. *J Clin Oncol*, **17**(3), 1061−70.

Eaton, L. (2004) *Ethics and the Business of Bioscience*, Electronic edn, Stanford University Press, Palo Alto, CA, USA.

Effros, R.B. (2003) Genetic alterations in the ageing immune system: Impact on infection and cancer. *Mechanisms of Ageing and Development*, **124**, 71−7.

Ehrke, M.J. (2003) Immunomodulation in cancer therapeutics. *International Immunopharmacology*, **451**, 1−15.

Ellis, L.M. (2005) Bevacizumab. *Nature Review Drug Discovery*, (Suppl S8−S9), S8−S9.

Entwistle, V., Tritter, J. and Calnan, M. (2002) Researching experiences of cancer: The importance of methodology. *European Journal of Cancer Care*, **11**, 232−7.

European Community (1998) In vitro diagnostic directive. Directive 98/79/EC, 7 Dec.

European Group for Tumor Markers (EGTM) (1999) Consensus recommendations. *Anticancer Res*, **19**, 2785−820. http://egtm.web.uni-muenchen.de/index2.html/ (Accessed Oct 2002).

European Union (2001) Directive 2001/20/EC. The Official Journal of the European Communities.

Evans, D. and Evans, M. (1996) A Recent Proposal: Ethical review of Clinical research, John Wiley & Sons, Chichester.

Faivre, S., Djelloul, S., Raymond, E. *et al.* (2006) New paradigms in anticancer therapy: Targeting multiple signalling pathways with kinase inhibitors. *Semin Oncol*, **33**(4), 407–20.

Fallowfield, L. (1990) *Quality of Life: The Missing Measurement in Health Care*, Souvenir Press, London.

Farol, L.T. and Hymes, K.B. (2004) Bexarotene: A clinical review. *Expert Rev Anticancer Ther*, **4**(2), 180–88.

Ferrajoli, A., Faderi, S. and Keating, M.J. (2006) Monoclonal antibodies in chronic lymphocytic leukemia. *Expert Review Anticancer Therapy*, **6**, 1231–38.

Fertig, D.L. and Hayes, D.F. (2001) Considerations in using tumour markers: What the psycho-oncologist needs to know. *Psycho-Oncology*, **10**, 370–9.

Fielding, J. and Phenow, K. (1988) Health effects of involuntary smoking. *New England Journal of Medicine*, **319**, 1452–60.

Finlay, G.J., Atwell, G.J., Baquley, B.C. *et al.* (1999) Inhibition of the action of the topo-isomerase II poison amsacrine by simple aniline derivatives: Evidence for drug-protein interactions. *Oncol Res*, **11**(6), 249–54.

Fleisher, M., Dnistrian, A.M., Sturgeon, C.M., Lamerz, R. and Wittliff, J.L. (2002) Practice guidelines and recommendations for use of tumor markers in the clinic. In: *Tumor Markers: Physiology, Pathobiology, Technology and Clinical Applications* (eds E.P. Diamandis, H. Fritsche, M.K. Schwartz and D.W. Chan), AACC Press, Chicago, 33–63.

Folkman, J. (1992) The role of angiogenesis in tumour growth. *Seminar Cancer Biology*, **3** (2), 65–71.

Folkman, J., Browder, T. and Palmblad, J. (2001) Angiogenesis research:guidelines for translation to clinical application. *Thrombosis and Haemostasis*, **8**, 23–33.

Foran, J.M. (2002) Antibody-based therapy of non-Hodgkin's lymphoma. *Best Practice and Research in Clinical Haematology*, **15**, 449–65.

Foster, C., Evans, D.G., Eeles, R. *et al.* (2002) Predictive testing for BRCA1/2: Attributes, risk perception and management in a multi-centre clinical cohort. *Br J Cancer*, **86**, 1209–6.

Foster, Claire (2001) *Ethics of Medical Research on Humans*, Cambridge University Press, Port Chester, NY, USA.

Fracasso, G., Bellisola, G., Cingarlini, S. *et al.* (2002) Anti-tumour effects of toxins targeted to the prostate specific membrane antigen. *The Prostate*, **53**, 9–23.

Franceschi, C., Bonafe, M. and Valensin, S. (2000) Human immunosenescence: The prevailing of innate immunity, the failing of colotypic immunity, and the filling of immunological space. *Vaccine*, **18**, 1717–20.

Frauwirth, K.A. and Thompson, C.B. (2002) Activation and inhibition of lymphocytes by co-stimulation. *J Clinical Investigation*, **109**, 295-9.

Freebairn, A.J.E., Last, A.T.J. and Illidge, T.M. (2001) Trastuzumab: Designer drug or fashionable fad? *Clinical Oncology*, **13**, 427–33.

Gabriel, J. (2001) Cancer: Health promotion, early detection and staging. In: *Oncology Nursing in Practice* (ed J.Gabriel), Whurr Publishers, London.

Gamba-Vitalo, C., Blair, O.C., Tritton, T.R. *et al.* (1987) Cytotoxicity and differentiating actions of adriamycin in WEHI-3B D+ leukaemia cells. *Leukemia*, **1**(3), 188–97.

Gandhi, V. and Plunkett, W. (1994) Evolution of the arabinosides and the pharmacology of fludarabine. *Drugs*, **47**(Suppl 6), 30–8.

Gardiner-Garden, M. and Frommer, M. (1987) CpG islands in vertebrate genomes. *J Mol. Biol*, **196**, 261−82.

Gibson, T.B., Ranganathan, A. and Grothey, A. (2006) Randomized phase III trial results of panitumumab, a fully human anti-epidermal growth factor receptor monoclonal antibody, in metastatic colorectal cancer. *Clinical Colorectal Cancer*, **6**(1), 29−31.

Gillis, C. (1978) The epidemiology of human cancers. In: *Oncology for Nurses and Health Care Professionals, Vol 1, Pathology, Diagnosis and Treatment* (ed P. Pritchard), Harper & Row, London.

Ginaldi, L., Loreta, M.F., Corsi, M.P., Modesti, M. and DeMartinis, M. (2001) Immunosenescence and infectious diseases. *Microbes and Infection*, **3**, 851−7.

Girard, M.P., Osmoanove, S.K. and Kieny, M.P. (2006) A review of vaccine research and development: The human immunodeficiency virus. *Vaccine*, **24**(19), 4062−81.

Glaser, B. and Strauss, A. (1967) *The Discovery of Grounded Theory: Strategies for Qualitative Research*, Aldine Publishing Company, New York.

Glover, D. (1999) Fully human monoclonal antibodies come to fruition. *Scrip Magazine*, May, 16−19.

Goldberg, D. and Williams, P. (1988) *A User's Guide to the General Health Questionnaire*, NFER-Nelson, Windsor.

Gollob, J.A., Wilhelm, S., Carter, C. and Kelley, S.L. (2006) Role of Raf kinase in cancer: Therapeutic potential of targeting the Raf/MEK/ERK signal transduction pathway. *Semin Oncol*, **33**(4), 392−406.

Goodin, R.E (1995) Utility and the good. In: *A Companion to Ethics*. Blackwell, Oxford.

Gorczynsky, R.M. and Stanley, J. (2006) *Problem-Based Immunology*, Elsevier, Philadelphia.

Govindan, R., Natale, R., Wade, J. *et al.* (2006) Efficacy and safety of gefininib in chemonaive patients with advanced non-small cell lung cancer treated in an Expanded Access Programme. *Lung Cancer*, **53**(3), 331−7.

Graham, J., Ramirez, A., Love, S., Richards, M. and Burgess, C. (2002) Stressful life experiences and risk of relapse of breast cancer: Observational cohort study. *BMJ*, **324**(7351), 1420.

Green, M.C., Murray, J.L. and Hortobagi, G N. (2000) Monoclonal antibody therapy of solid tumours. *Cancer Treatment Reviews*, **26**, 269−86.

Greenhalgh, T. (2001) *How to Read a Paper: The Basics of Evidenced Based Medicine*, BMJ Books, London.

Grusenmeyer, P.A. and Wong Y.N. (2007) Interpreting the economic literature in oncology. *J Clin Ducol*, **25** (2), 196−2002.

Gulbahce, H.E., Brown, C.A., Wick, M., Segall, M. and Jessurun, J. (2003) Graft-vs-host disease after organ transplant. *American J Clinical Pathology*, **119**(4), 568−73.

Gura, T. (2002) Magic bullets hit the target. *Nature*, **417**, 584−6.

Gusella, J.F. and MacDonald, M.E. (1993) Hunting for Huntington's disease. *Mol Genet Med*, **3**, 139−58.

Hainsworth, J.D. (2000) Monoclonal antibody therapy in lymphoid malignancies. *The Oncologist*, **5**, 376−84.

Hait, W.N. (2001) The prognostic and predictive values of ECD-HER-2. *Clinical Cancer Research*, **7**, 2601−4.

Hall, A.G. and Tilby, M.J. (1992) Mechanism of action of and modes of resistance to alkylating agents used in the treatment of haematological malignancies. *Blood Rev*, **6**(3), 163−73.

Halloran, C.M., Ghaneh, P., Neoptolemos, J.P. and Costello, E. (2000) Gene therapy for pancreatic cancer – current and prospective strategies. *Surgical Oncology*, **9**, 181–91.

Hammersley, M. and Atkinson, P. (1983) *Ethnography: Principles and Practice*, Tavistock, London.

Hammond, M.E., Fitzgibbons, P.L., Compton, C.C., Grignon, D.J., Page, D.L., Fielding, L.P. *et al.* (2000) College of American Pathologists Conference XXXV: solid tumor prognostic factors – which, how and so what? Summary document and recommendations for implementation. Cancer Committee and Conference Participants. *Arch Pathol Lab Med*, **124**(7), 958–65.

Hammond, M.E., Taube, S.E. (2002) Issues and barriers to development of clinically useful tumor markers: a development pathway proposal. *Semin Oncol*, **29**(3), 213–21.

Hampel, H., Sweet, K., Westman, J.A., Offit, K. and Eng, C. (2004) Referral for cancer genetics consultation: A review and compilation of risk assessment criteria. *Journal of Medical Genetics*, **41**, 81–91.

Hanahan, D. and Folkman, J. (1996) Patterns and emerging mechanisms of the angiogenic switch during tumorigenesis. *Cell*, **86**(3), 353–64.

Hanahan, D. and Weinberg, R.A. (2000) The hallmarks of cancer. *Cell*, **100**(1), 57–70.

Hansen, M.F. and Cavenee, W.K. (1988) Tumor suppressors: Recessive mutations that lead to cancer. *Cell*, **53**, 173–4.

Harries, M. and Smith, I. (2002) The development and clinical use of trastuzumab (Herceptin). *Endocrine-Related Cancer*, **9**, 75–85.

Harris, M. (2004) Monoclonal antibodies as therapeutic agents for cancer. *Lancet Oncology*, **5**, 292–302.

Harrocopus, C. and Myers, C. (1996) *Stoma Care Nursing*, Edward Arnold, London.

Hartman, J.T. and Lipp, H.P. (2006) Camptothecin and podophyllotoxin derivatives: Inhibitors of topoisomerase I and II, mechanisms of action, pharmacokinetics and toxicity profile. *Drug Saf*, **29**(3), 209–30.

Hausen, L. (1991) Viruses in human cancers. *Science*, **254**, 1167–73.

Hayes, D.F., Trock, B. and Harris, A.L. (1998) Assessing the clinical impact of prognostic factors: When is "statistically significant" clinical useful. *Breast Cancer Research and Treatment*, **52**, 305–19.

Heald, P., Mehlmauer, M., Martin, A.G. *et al.* (2003) Topical bexarotene therapy for patients with refractory or persistent early stage cutaneous T cell lymphoma: Results of the phase III clinical trial. *J Am Acad Dermatol*, **49**(5), 801–15.

Hecht, S.M. (2000) Bleomycin: New perspectives on the mechanism of action. *J Nat Prod*, **63**(1), 158–68.

Henson, D.E., Fielding, L.P., Grignon, D.J., Page, D.L., Hammond, M.E., Nash, G. *et al.* (1995) College of American Pathologists Conference XXVI on clinical relevance of prognostic markers in solid tumors. Summary. Members of the Cancer Committee. *Arch Pathol Lab Med*, **119**(12), 1109–12.

Hermansson, M., Nistér, M., Betsholtz, C. *et al.* (1988) Endothelial cell hyperplasia in human glioblastoma: Coexpression of mRNA for platelet-derived growth factor (PDGF) B chain and PDGF receptor suggests autocrine growth stimulation. *Proceedings of the National Academy of Sciences of the United States of America*, **85**(20), 7748–52.

Hirsch, J. (2006) An anniversary for cancer chemotherapy. *JAMA*, **296**(12), 1518–20.

Hitt, R., Lopez-Pousa, A., Martinez-Trufero, J. *et al.* (2005) Phase III study comparing cisplatin plus fluorouracil to paclitaxel, cisplatin and fluorouracil induction chemotherapy followed by chemoradiotherapy in locally advanced head and neck cancer. *J Clin Oncol*, **23**(34), 8636—45.

Holt, L.J., Enever, C., deWildt, R.M.T and Tomlinson, I.M. (2000) The use of recombinant antibodies in proteomics. *Current Opinions in Biotechnology*, **11**, 445—9.

Hong, V. and Erusalimsky, J.D. (2002) Comparison of the pharmacological mechanisms involved in the platelet lowering actions of anagrelide and hydroxyurea: A review. *Platelets*, **13**(7), 381—6.

Hood, L.E. (2003) Chemotherapy in the elderly: Supportive measures for chemotherapy-induced myelotoxicity. *Clinical J Oncol Nursing*, **7**(2), 185—90.

Horton-Taylor, D. (2001) Cancer and epidemiology. In: *Cancer Nursing Care in Context* (eds J. Corner and C. Bailey), Blackwell Publishing, Oxford.

Howell, A., Cuzick, J. and Baum, M. (2005) Results of the ATAC (Arimidex, Tamoxifen Alone or in Combination) trial after completion of 5 years adjuvant treatment for breast cancer. *Lancet*, **365**(9453), 60—2. http://www.nci.nih.gov/newscenter/edrn (Accessed Nov. 2002).

Hudson, P.J. and Souriau, C. (1993) Engineered antibodies. *Nature Medicine*, **9**, 129—34.

Human Tissue Act (2004)

International Human Genome Sequencing Consortium (2004) Finishing the euchromatic sequence of the human genome. *Nature*, **431**, 931—45.

Itsuro, J. (2007) 3. Imatinib therapy in chronic myelogenous leukaemia. *Internal Med*, **46**(2), 95—7.

Jenkins, V. and Fallowfield, L. (2000) Reasons for accepting or declining to participate in randomised clinical trials for cancer therapy. *British Journal of Cancer*, **82**(11), 1783—88.

Jordan, M.A. and Wilson, L. (2004) Microtubules as a target for anticancer drugs. *Nature Reviews Cancer*, **4**, 253—65.

Jorde, L.B., Carey, J.C., Bamshad, M.J. and White, R.L. (2000) Cancer genetics. In: *Medical Genetics* (ed W. Schmitt), 2nd cdn, Mosby, Inc., St Louis, pp. 221—38.

Juweid, M.E. (2002) Radioimmunotherapy of B-cell non-Hodgkin's lymphoma: From clinical trials to clinical practice. *Journal of Nuclear Medicine*, **43**, 1507—29.

Kallioniemi, A., Kallioniemi, O.P., Sudar, D. *et al.* (1992) Comparative genomic hybridisation for molecular cytogenetic analysis of solid tumours. *Science*, **258**, 818 21.

Kamen, B. (1997) Folate and antifolate pharmacology. *Semin Oncol*, **24**(5 supl. 18), S18-30—S18-39.

Kashiwagi, H. and Uchida, K. (2000) Genome-wide profiling of gene amplification and deletion in cancer. *Hum Cell*, **13**, 135—41.

Kennedy, I. and Grubb, A. (2000) *Medical Law, Third Edition*. Butterworths, London.

Kerbel, R. and Folkman, J. (2002) Clinical translation of angiogenesis inhibitors. *Nat Rev Cancer*, **2**(10), 727—39.

Kerkela, R., Grazette, L., Yacobi, R. *et al.* (2006) *Research Medicine*;advance online publication, 23 July.

Kerr, D. (2003) Clinical development of gene therapy for colorectal cancer. *Nat Rev Cancer*, **3**, 615—22.

Khan, J., Bittner, M.L., Chen, Y., Meltzer, P.S. and Trent, J.M. (1999) DNA microarray technology: The anticipated impact on the study of human disease. *Biochim Biophys Acta*, **1423**, M17—28.

Khatcheressian, J.L., Wolff, A.C., Smith, T.J. *et al.* (2006) ASCO 2006 update of the breast cancer follow-up and management guidelines in the adjuvant setting. *J Clin Oncol*, **24**, 5091—7.

Kinzler, K.W. and Vogelstein, B. (1996) Lessons from hereditary colorectal cancer. *Cell*, **87**, 159–70.

Kirkbride, K.C. and Blobe, G.C. (2003) Inhibition of the TGFb signalling pathway as means of cancer immunotherapy. *Expert Opinion Biological Therapy*, **3**(2), 251–61.

Klapdor, R., Aronsson, A.C., Duffy, M.J. *et al.* (1999) Tumor markers in gastrointestinal cancers: EGTM recommendations. *Anticancer Res*, **19**, 2811–15.

Klasa, R.J., Meyer, R.M., Shustik, C. *et al.* (2002) Randomised phase III study of fludarabine phosphate versus cyclophosphamide, vincristine and prednisolone in patients with recurrent low grade Non-Hodgkin's lymphoma previously treated with an alkylating agent or alkylator containing regimen. *J Clin Oncol*, **20**(24), 4649–54.

Knudson, A.G., Jr (1971) Mutation and cancer: Statistical study of retinoblastoma. *Proc Natl Acad Sci USA*, **68**, 820–3.

Koch, T. (1995) Interpretive approaches in nursing research: The influence of Husserl and Heidegger. *Journal of Advanced Nursing*, **24**, 827–36.

Koch, T. (1996) Implementation of a hermeneutic inquiry in nursing: Philosophy, rigour and representation. *Journal of Advanced Nursing*, **24**, 174–84.

Köhler, G. and Milstein, C. (1975) Continuous culture of fused cells secreting specific antibody of predefined specificity. *Nature*, **256**, 495–7.

Kornberg, R.D. and Lorch, Y. (1999) Twenty-five years of the nucleosome, fundamental particle of the eukaryote chromosome. *Cell*, **98**, 285–94.

Kothari, M.L. and Mehta, L. (2002) Bipolar hermaphroditism of somatic cell as the basis of its being and becoming: Celldom appreciated. *J. Postgrad Med*, **48**, 232–7.

Kovaiou, R.D. and Grubeck-Loebenstein, B. (2006) Age-associated changes within CD4+ T cells. *Immunology Letter*, **107**(1), 8–14.

Kramer, B.S. and Klausner, R.D. (1997) Grappling with cancer – defeatism versus the reality of progress. *N Engl J Med*, **337**, 931–4.

Kricka, L.J. (2000) Interferences in immunoassay – still a threat. [Editorial]. *Clin Chem*, **46**, 1037–8.

Kubota, Y., Ohji, H., Itoh, K., Sasagawa, I. and Nakada, T. (2001) Changes in cellular imunity during chemotherapy for testicular cancer. *International Journal of Urology*, **8**, 604–8.

Kuroki, M., Ueno, A., Mastumoto, H. *et al.* (2002) Significance of tumour-associated antigens in the diagnosis and therapy of cancer: An overview. *Anticancer Research*, **22**, 4255–64.

Kyle, R.A. (1975) Multiple myeloma: Review of 869 cases. *Mayo Clin Proc*, **50**, 29–40.

Lal, A., Lash, A.E., Altschul, S.F., Velculescu, V., Zhang, L., McLendon, R.E. *et al.* (1999) A public database for gene expression in human cancers. *Cancer Res*, **59**(21), 5403–7.

Lamerz, R., Albrecht, W., Bialk, P. *et al.* (1999) Tumour markers in germ cell cancers: EGTM recommendations. *Anticancer Res*, **19**, 2795–8. British Association of Urological Surgeons. *BJU Int*, **84**, 987–1014.

Le Chevalier, T., Brisgand, D., Douillard, J.Y. *et al.* (1994) Randomised study of vinorelbine and cisplatin versus vindesine and cisplatin versus vinorelbine alone in advanced non-small cell lung cancer: Results of a European multicenter trial including 612 patients. *J Clin Oncol*, **12**, 360–7.

Leitner, W.W., Ying, H. and Restifo, N.P. (2000) DNA and RNA-based vaccines: Principles. Progress and prospects (Review). *Vaccines*, **18**, 765–7.

Leonard, J.P. and Link, B.K. (2002) Immunotherapy of non-Hodgkin's lymphoma with hLL2 (Epratuzumab, an anti-CD-22 monoclonal antibody) and HUD10 (Apolizumab). *Seminars in Oncology*, **29**(Suppl 2), 81–6.

Levings, M.K., Bacchetta, R., Schultz, U. and Roncarolo, M.G. (2002) The role of IL-10 and TGF-beta in the differentiation and effector function of T regulatory cells. *Int Arch Allergy Immmulogy*, **129**(4), 263—76.

Lewin, B. (2003) *Genes VIII*, Oxford University Press, Oxford.

Lind, J., Hagan, L. (2000) Bladder and kidney cancer. In: Greonwald, S., Frogge, M.,, Goodman, M., Yarbo, C. (eds), *Cancer Nursing: Principles and Practice*, 5th edn, Jones and Bartlett, Boston, MA.

Lippert, B. (1999) *Cisplatin: Chemistry and Biochemistry of a Leading Anticancer Drug*, John Wiley and Sons, New York.

LoBiondo-Wood, G. and Haber, J. (1998) *Nursing Research: Methods, Critical Appraisal, and Utilization*, 4th edn, Mosby, London.

Locker, G.Y., Hamilton, S., Harris, J. *et al.* (2006) ASCO 2006 update of recommendations for the use of tumor markers in gastrointestinal cancer. *J Clin Oncol*, **24**, 313—27.

Loeb, L.A. (1994) Microsatellite instability: Marker of a mutator phenotype in cancer. *Cancer Res*, **54**, 5059—63.

Lollini, P.L. and Forni, G. (2003) Cancer immunoprevention: Tracking down persistent tumour antigens. *Trends in Imunology*, **24**(2), 62—6.

Lords, J.M., Butcher, S., Killampali, V., Lascelles, D. and Salmon, M. (2001) Neutrophil ageing and immunescence. *Mechanisms Ageing and Development*, **122**, 1521—35.

Lundqvist, A. and Pisa, P. (2002) Gene-modified dendritic cells and immunotherapy against cancer. *Medical Oncology*, **19**(4), 197—211.

Lutz, J. and Heemann, U. (2003) Tumours after kidney transplantation. *Current Opinion Urology*, **13**(2), 105—9.

Lynch, H. and Alban,W. (1984) Genetic biomarkers and the Heieck control of breast cancer. *Cancer Genetics and Cytogenetics*, **13**, 43—92.

Macleod, K. (2000) Tumor suppressor genes. *Curr Opin Genet Dev*, **10**, 81—93.

Madsen, S. *et al.* (2002) Attitudes towards clinical trials. *Journal of Internal Medicine*, **251**, 156—68.

Magdelenat, H. (1992) Tumour markers in oncology: Past, present and future. *Journal of Immunological Methods*, **150**, 133—43.

Malaguarnera, L., Ferlito, L., Di Mauro, S. *et al.* (2001) Immunoscnescence and cancer: a review. *Arch Gerontol Geriate*, **32**(2) 77—93.

Marieb, E.N. and Hoehn K (2007) *Human Anatomy and Physiology, Chapter 21*, 7th edn, Pearson Education, London.

Marks, C. and Marks, J.D. (1996) Phage libraries: A new route to clinically useful antibodies. *New England Journal of Medicine*, **335**, 730—3.

Marks, V. (2002) False-Positive immunoassay results: A multicenter survey of erroneous immunoassay results from assays of 74 analytes in 10 donors from 66 laboratories in seven countries. *Clin Chem* **48**, 2008—16.

Marth, C., Trope, C., Vergote, I.B. and Kritensen, G.B. (1998) Ten year results of a randomised trial comparing cisplatin with cisplatin and cyclophosphamide in advanced, suboptimally debulked ovarian cancer. *Eur J Cancer*, **34**(8), 1175—80.

Mays, N and Pope, C. (1995) Qualitative research: Rigour and qualitative research. *BMJ*, **311**, 109—12.

McHugh, R.S. and Shevach, E.M. (2002) The role of suppressor T cells in regulation of immune responses. *Allergy Clinical Immunology*, **110**(5), 693—702.

McLemore, M.R. (2006) Gardasil: Introducing the new human papilomavirus vaccine. *Clinical Journal of Oncology Nursing*, **10**(5), 559—60.

Mead, G.M. (1995) Chemotherapy for solid tumours: Routine treatment not yet justified. *BMJ*, **310**, 246−7.

Medical Research Council Brain Tumour Working Party (2001) Randomised trial of procarbazine, lomustine and vincristine in the adjuvant treatment of high grade astrocytoma. A Medical Research Council Trial. *J Clin Oncol*, **19**(2), 509−18.

Medicines for Human Use (Clinical Trials) Regulations (2004) The Stationery Office Ltd, London.

Menard, S., Pupa, S.M., Campiglio, M. and Tagliabue, E. (2003) Biologic and therapeutic role of HER2 in cancer. *Oncogene*, **22**, 6570−8.

Mendelsohn, J. (2001) The epidermal growth factor receptor as a target for cancer therapy. *Endocrine-Related Cancer*, **8**, 3−9.

Mental Capacity Act (2005).

Miles, L.E.H. and Hales, C.N. (1968) Labelled antibodies and immunological assay systems. *Nature*, **219**, 186−9.

Miller, R.A. (1996) The ageing immune system: Primer and prospectus. *Science*, **273**, 70−4.

Modjtahedi, H. and Dean, C. (1994) The receptor for EGF and its ligands: Expression, prognostic value and target for therapy in cancer (Review). *International Journal of Oncology*, **4**, 277−96.

Modjtahedi, H., Hickish, T. and Nicolson, M. *et al.* (1996) A phase I trial and tumour localization of the anti-EGFR antibody ICR62 in head and neck or lung cancer. *British Journal of Cancer*, **73**, 228−35.

Moingeon, P. (2001) Cancer vaccines (review). *Vaccine*, **19**, 1305−26.

Molassiotis, A, Gibson, F. and Kelly, D. *et al.* (2006) A systematic review of worldwide cancer nursing research. *Cancer Nursing*, **29**(6), 431−40.

Molina, R., Duffy, M.J. and Aronsson, A.C. *et al.* (1999) Tumor markers in breast cancer: EGTM recommendations. *Anticancer Res*, **19**, 2803−5.

Morgan, R.A., Dudley, M.E. and Wunderlich, J.R. *et al.* (2006) Cancer regression in patients after transfer of genetically engineered lymphocytes. *Science*, **314**, 126−9.

Morimoto, Y., Tanaka, Y. and Itoh, T. *et al.* (2002) Spontanous necrosis of hepatocellular carcinoma: A case report. *Dig Surg*, **19**, 413−18.

Motzer, R.J., Hutson, T.E. and Tomczak, P. *et al.* (2007) Sunitinib versus interferon alfa in metastatic renal cell carcinoma. *N Engl J Med*, **356**(2), 115−24.

Motzer, R.J., Sheinfeld, J. and Mazumdar, M. (2000) Paclitaxel, ifosfamide and cisplatin second line therapy for patients with relapsed testicular germ cell cancer. *J Clin Oncol*, **18**, 2413−18.

Muggia, F.M. and Fojo, T. (2004) Platinums: Extending their therapeutic spectrum. *J Chemother*, **16**(Suppl 4), 77−82.

Munhall, P. (1982) Nursing philosophy and nursing research: in apposition or opposition. *Nursing Research*, **31**(3), 176−7.

Murphy, A. and Cowman, S. (2006) Research priorites of oncology nurses in the Republic of Ireland. *Cancer Nursing*, **29**(4), 283−90.

Nagle, A., Hur, W. and Gray, N.S. (2006) Antimitotic agents of natural origin. *Curr Drug Targets*, **7**(3), 305−26.

Naito, Y., Saito, K., Shiiba, K. *et al.* (1998) CD8+ T cells infiltrated within cancer cell nests as a prognostic factor in human colorectal cancer. *Cancer Research*, **58**, 3491−94.

Nakano, O., Sato, M., Naito, Y. *et al.* (2001) Proliferation activity of itratumoural CD8+ T-lymphocytes as a prognostic factor in human renal cell carcinoma: clinicopathogenic demonstration of antitumour immunity. *Cancer Research*, **61**, 5132−36.

Nakayama, Y., Nagashima, N., Minagawa, N. *et al.* (2002) Relationship between tumur associated macrophages and clinicopathological factors in patients with colorectal cancer. *Anticancer Research*, **22**, 4291−96.

Natali, P.G., Nicotra, M.R., Bigotti, A. *et al.* (1989) Selective changes in expression of HLA class I polymorphic determinants in human tumours. *Proceeding National Academy Sciences*, **86**, 6719−23.

National Cancer Research Network (NCRN) (2001) *Newsletter*, November.

National Institute for Clinical Excellence (NICE) (2003) *Improving Supportive and Palliative Care for Adults with Cancer*. NICE, London.

National Institute for Health and Clinical Excellence (2006) *Docetaxel for the Treatment of Hormone Refractory Metastatic Prostate Cancer*. NICE Technology Appraisal 101. NICE, London.

National Institute for Health and Clinical Excellence (2007) *Bevacizumab and Cetuximab for the Treatment of Metastatic Colorectal Cancer*. NICE Technology Appraisal 118. NICE, London.

National Institute for Clinical Excellence (NICE) (2005) *Improving Outcomes Guidance for People with Skin Tumours Including Melanoma*. NICE, London.

National Translational Cancer Research Network (2002) Mission Statement. http://www.ntrac.org.uk (Accessed 25 Jan 2007).

NCAB Working Group on Biomedical Technology (2005) Report to National Cancer Advisory Borad. http://deainfo.nci.nih.gov/advisory/ncab/sub-bt/NCABReport_Feb05.pdf (Accesed April 2007).

NCAB Working Group on Biomedical Technology (2005) Report to National Cancer Advisory Borad. http://deainfo.nci.nih.gov/advisory/ncab/sub-bt/NCABReport_Feb05.pdf (Accesed April 2007).

NCI (2005) *Report to National Cancer Advisory Board*. NCAB Working Group on Biomedical Technology.

NCI *Dictionary of Cancer Terms*. http://www.cancer.gov/templates/db_alpha.aspx? (Accessed Nov 2006).

NCRI (2004) *3 Year Progress Report 2001−2004*. National Cancer Research Institute, London.

Needle, M.N. (2002) Safety experience with IMC-225, an anti-epidermal growth factor receptor antibody. *Seminars in Oncology*, **29**(Suppl 14), 55−60.

Nencioni, A., Grunebach, F., Patrone, F. *et al.* (2007) Proteosome inhibitors: Antitumour effects and beyond. *Leukemia*, **21**(1), 30−6.

Newell, D., Gescher, A., Hartland, S. *et al.* (1987) N-methyl antitumour agents. A distinct class of anticancer drugs. *Cancer Chemother Pharmacol*, **19**(2), 91−102.

Nicholson, R.I., Gee, J.M.W. and Harper, M.E. (2001) EGFR and cancer prognosis. *European Journal of Cancer*, **37**, S9−S15.

Norum, J. (2006) The cost effectiveness issue of adjuvant trastuzumab in early breast cancer. *Expert Opinion Pharmacotherapy*, **7**(12), 1217−625.

Nursing Midwifery Council (2004) *Code of Professional Conduct: Standards for Conduct, Performance and Ethics*. NMC, London.

Nursing Midwifery Council (2006) *Research and Audit − A-Z advice sheet*. NMC, London.

Nustad, K., Bast, R.C. Jr, Brien, T.J. *et al.* (1996) Specificity and affinity of 26 monoclonal antibodies against the CA 125 antigen: first report from the ISOBM TD-1 workshop. International Society for Oncodevelopmental Biology and Medicine. *Tumour Biol*, **17**(4), 196−219.

O'Mahony, M. (2001) Women's lived experience of breast biopsy: A phenomenological study. *Journal of Clinical Nursing*, **10**, 512−20.

O'Shaughnessy, J., Miles, D., Vukelja, S. *et al*. (2002) Superior survival with capecitabine plus docetaxel combination therapy in anthracycline-pretreated patients with advanced breast cancer: Phase III trial results. *J Clin Oncol*, **20**(12), 2812−3.

Ohno, S., Inagawa, H., Soma, G.I., and Nagasue, N. (2002) Role of tumour-associated macrophages in malignant tumours: Should the location of the infiltrated macrophages be taken into account during evaluation. *Anticancer Research*, **22**, 4269−76.

Ozanne B, Richards, C.S., Hendler, F., Burns D. and Gusterson B. (1986) Over-expression of the EGF receptor is a hallmark of squamous cell carcinomas, *J.Pathol*: **149**, 9−14.

Pagliargo, L.C., Liu, B., Munker, R. *et al*. (1998) Humanized M195 monoclonal antibody conjugate to recombinant Gelonin: an anti-CD33 immunotoxin with antileukemic activity. *Clinical Cancer Research*, **4**, 1971−6.

Paley, J. (1997) Husserl, phenomenology and nursing. *Journal of Advanced Nursing*, **26**, 187−93.

Palmer, A. (2001) Understanding radiotherapy and its applications. In: *Oncology Nursing in Practice* (ed J. Gabriel), Whurr, London.

Pangalis, G.A., Dimopoulou, M.N., Angelopoulou, M.K. *et al*. (2001) Campath-1H (Anti-CD520 monoclonal antibody therapy in lymphoproliferative disorders. *Medical Oncology*, **18**, 99−107.

Papac, R.J. (1998) Spontaneous regression of cancer: possible mechanisms. *In Vivo*, **12**(6), 571−8.

Parahoo, K. (1997) *Nursing Research: Principles, Process and Issues*. Macmillan Press Ltd, London.

Pardal, R., Clarke, M.F. and Morrison, S.J. (2003) Applying the principles of stem-cell biology to cancer. *Nature Rev Cancer*, **3**, 895−902.

Parfitt, K. (ed) (2005) *Martindale. The Complete Drug Reference*, 34th edn, Pharmaceutical Press, London.

Pardoll, D.M. (1998) Cancer vaccines. *Nature Medicine*, **4** (suppl 5), 525−31.

Parkin, D.M. (2001) Global cancer statistics in the year 2000. *Lancet Oncology*, **2**(9), 533−43.

Paschen, A., Mendez, R.M., Jimenez, P. *et al*. (2003) Complete loss of HLA Class I antigen expression on melanoma cells: A result of successive mutational events. *International J Cancer*, **103**, 759−69.

Pastan, I., Hassan, R., Fitzgerald, D.J. and Keritman, R.J. (2006) Immunotoxin therapy of cancer. *Nature Review Cancer*, **6**, 559−65.

Patel, A.A. and Steitz, J.A. (2003) Splicing double: Insights from the second spliceosome. *Nature Rev. Mol. Cell Biol*, **4**, 960.

Pavlou, A.K. and Belsey, M.J. (2005) The therapeutic antibodies market to 2008. *Eur J Pharmaceutics and Biopharmaceutics*, **59**, 389−96.

Pinedo, H. and Salmon, D. [2000] Translational research. The role of VEGF in tumour angiogenesis. *The Oncologist*, [Suppl1], 1−2.

Ponder, B.A. (2001) Cancer genetics. *Nature*, **411**, 336−41.

Popay, J. and Williams G. (1998) Qualitative research and evidence-based healthcare. *Journal of the Royal Society of Medicine*, **91**(35), 32−7.

Pronzato, P., Landucci, M., Vaira, F. *et al*. (1994) Carboplatin and etoposide as outpatient treatment of advanced non-small cell lung cancer. *Chemotherapy*, **40**(2), 144−8.

Rabson, A., Roitt, I.M. and Delves, P.J. (2005) *Really Essential Medical Immunology*, 2nd edn, Blackwell Publishing, Oxford.

Rader, M. (2006) Granulocyte colony-stimulating factor use in patients with chemotherapy-induced neutropenia: Clinical and economic benefits. *Oncology*, **20**(Suppl 5),16−21.

Rai, K.R., Freter, C.E., Mercier, R.J. *et al.* (2002) Alemtuzumab in previously treated chronic lymphocytic leukemia patients who also received fludarabine. *Journal of Clinical Oncology*, **20**, 3891−7.

Ramirez, A., Craig, T., Watson, J. *et al.* (1989) Stress and relapse of breast cancer. *BMJ*, **298**, 291−3.

Rang, H.P., Dale, M.M., Ritter, J.M. and Moore, P.K. (2003) *Pharmacology*, 5th edn, Churchill Livingstone, Edinburgh.

Ray-Coquard, I., Borg, C., Bachelot, T. *et al.* (2003) Baseline and early lymphopenia predict for the risk of febrile neutropenia after chemotherapy. *British Journal of Cancer*, **88**, 181−6.

Reichardt, P., vonMinckwitz, G., Thuss-Patience, P.C. *et al.* (2003) Multicentre phase II study of oral capecitabine ("Xeloda") in patients with metastatic breast cancer relapsing after treatment with a taxane-containing therapy. *Ann Oncol*, **14**(8), 1227−33.

Reik, W. and Walter, J. (2001) Genomic imprinting: parental influence on the genome. *Nat Rev Genet*, **2**, 21−32.

Reya, T., Morrison, S.J., Clarke, M.F. and Weissman, I.L. (2001) Stem cells, cancer, and cancer stem cells. *Nature*, **414**, 105−11.

Rhee, I., Jair, K.W., Yen, R.W. *et al.* (2000) CpG methylation is maintained in human cancer cells lacking DNMT1. *Nature*, **404**, 1003−7.

Richard, L., Association of the British Pharmaceutical Industry (2006) http://www.bbcnews.co.uk/1/hi/London/England (Accessed Feb 2007).

Richards, M. (2006) *Network Development Programme (NDP) Update Session, October 2006*. Renaissance Hotel, Heathrow.

Richards, T.I. and Richards, L. (1990) *Manual for Mainframe NUD.IST Software Version 2.1*. Replee, Melbourne.

Richardson, A., Miller, M. and Potter, H. (2002) *Developing, Delivering and Evaluating Cancer Nursing Services. Building the Evidence Base.* King's College, London.

Rogowski, W. (2006) Genetic screening by DNA technology: A systematic review of health economic evidence. *Int J Technol Assess Health Care*, **22**, 327−7.

Romero, P., Pittet, M., Dutoit, V. *et al.* (2002) Therapeutic cancer vaccines based on molcularly defined human tumour antigens. *Vaccine*, **20**, A2−A7.

Ropponen, K.M., Eskelinen, M.J., Lipponen P.K., Alhava, E. and Kosma, V.M. (1997) Prognostic value of tumour infiltrating lymphocytes (TILs) in colorectal cancer. *Journal of Pathology*, **182**, 318−24.

Rosenberg, P., Andersson, H., Boman, K. *et al.* (2002) Randomized trial of single agent paclitaxel given weekly versus every three weeks and with peroral versus intravenous steroid premedication to patients with ovarian cancer previously treated with platinum. *Acta Oncol*, **41**(5), 418−24.

Royal College of Radiologists 'Clinical Oncology Information Network Guidelines on the management of prostate cancer (1999) A document for local expert groups in the United Kingdom preparing prostate management policy documents. British Association of Urological Surgeons. *BJU Int*, **84**, 987−1014.

Rubin, I. and Yarden, Y. (2001) The basic biology of HER-2. *Annals on Oncology*, **12**(Suppl 1) S3−S8.

Sabel, M.S. and Sondak, V.K. (2002) Melanoma vaccines: breakthrough or bust. *Cancer Investigation*, **20**, 1114–6.

Salgaller, M.L., Tjoa, B.A., Lodge, P.A. *et al.* (1998) Dendritic cell-based immunotherapy of prostate cancer. Critical ReviewTM. *Immunology*, **18**, 109–9.

Salkind, N. (2000) *Statistics for People Who Hate Statistics*. Sage Publications Inc. London.

Sambrook, J. and Russell, D.W. (2001) *Molecular Cloning: A Laboratory Manual*, 3rd edn, Cold Spring Harbor Laboratory Press, Cold Spring Harbour, NY.

Samson, D., Gaminara, E., Newland, A. *et al.* (1989) Infusion of vincristine and doxorubicin with oral dexamethasone as first line therapy for multiple myeloma. *Lancet*, **2**, 882–5.

Scadden, D.T. (2003) AIDS-related malignancies. *Annual Review Medicine*, **54**, 285–303.

Scheithauer, W., Kornek, G.V., Raderer, M. *et al.* (2003) Randomised multicentre phase II trial of two different schedules of capecitabine plus oxaliplatin as first line treatment in advanced colorectal cancer. *J Clin Oncol*, **21**(7), 1307–2.

Schiller, J.H., Harrington, D., Belani, C.P. *et al.* (2002) Comparison of four chemotherapy regimens for advanced non-small cell lung cancer. *N Eng J Med*, **346**(2), 92–8.

Schilsky, R.L. and Taube, S.E. (2002) Tumor markers as clinical cancer tests – are we there yet. *Semin Oncol*, **29**(3), 211–2.

Schrag, D. (2004) The price tag on progress-chemotherapy for colorectal cancer. *New England Journal of Medicine*, **351**, 317–9.

Scott, S.D. (1998) Rituximab: A new therapeutic monoclonal antibody for non-Hodgkin's lymphoma. *Cancer Practice*, **6**, 195–7.

Scottish Medicines Consortium (2005) *Cetuximab in Combination With Irinotecan for the Treatment of Patents With Epidermal Growth Factor (EGFR) Expressing Metastatic Colorectal Cancer After Failure of Irinotecan Including Cytotoxic Chemotherapy (155/05)*. SMC, Edinburgh.

Scottish Medicines Consortium (2005) *Docetaxel in combination with Prednisolone for the Treatment of Patients with Hormone Refractory Metastatic Prostate Cancer (209/05)*. SMC, Edinburgh

Scottish Medicines Consortium (2006) *Bortezomib as Monotherapy for the Treatment of Progressive Multiple Myeloma in Patients Who Have Received at Least One Prior Therapy and Who Have Already Undergone or Are Unsuitable for a Bone Marrow Transplant (302/06)*. SMC, Edinburgh.

Scottish Medicines Consortium (2006) *Mitotane 500mg Tablets (328/06)*. SMC, Edinburgh.

Semjonow, A., Albrecht, W., Bialk, P. *et al.* (1999) Tumour markers in prostate cancer: EGTM recommendations. *Anticancer Res*, **19**, 2799–801.

Sharkey, R.M. and Goldenberg, D.M. (2006) Targeted therapy of cancer: new prospects for antibodies and immunoconjugate. *CA Cancer J Clin*, **56**, 226–43.

Sheppard, C. (2001) Breast cancer. In: *Oncology Nursing in Practice* (ed J. Gabriel), Whurr, London.

Shih, T. and Lindley, C. (2006) Bevacizumab: An angiogenesis inhibitor for the treatment of solid malignancies. *Clin Ther*, **28**(11), 1779–802.

Shimada, H., Ochiai, T. and Nomura F. (2003) Titration of serum p53 antibodies in 1085 patients with various types of malignant tumours. *Cancer*, **97**, 682–9.

Sikora, K., Adrani, S., Koroltchouk, V. *et al.* (1999) Essential drugs for cancer therapy: A World Health Organisation consultation. *Ann Oncol*, **10**(4),385–90.

Sliwkowski, M.X., Lofgren, J.A., Lewis, G.D. *et al.* (1999) Nonclinical studies addressing the mechanism of action of trastuzumab (Herceptin). *Seminars in Oncology*, **26**(Suppl 12), 60–70.

Smith, I., Proctor, M., Gelber, R.D. *et al.* (2007) Two year follow up of trastuzumab after adjuvant chemotherapy in HER-2 positive breast cancer: A randomised controlled trial. *Lancet*, **369**(9555), 29–36.

Solana, R. and Mariani, E. (2000) NK and NK/T cells in human senescence. *Vaccine*, **18**, 1613–20.

Southern, E.M. (1975) Detection of specific sequences among DNA fragments separated by gel electrophoresis. *J Mol Biol*, **98**(3), 503–17.

Specific cancer: Melanoma skin cancer (2002) http://www.cancerhelp.org.uk/help/default. asp?page=3009 (Accessed 11 Feb 2007).

Specific cancers: Breast cancer (2002) http://www.cancerhelp.org.uk/help/default.asp? page=3284 (Accessed 11 Feb 2007).

Specific cancers: Colorectal (bowel) cancer (2002) http://www.cancerhelp.org.uk/ help/default.asp?page=2806 (Accessed 11 Feb 2007).

Specific cancers: Lung cancer (2002) http://www.cancerhelp.org.uk/help/default.asp? page=2964 (Accessed 11 Feb 2007).

Speck, L.M. and Tyring, S.K. (2006) Vaccines for the prevention of human papilomavirus infections. *Skin Therapy Letter*, **11**(6), 1–3.

Spiridon, C.I., Guinn, S. and Vitetta, E.S. (2004) A comparison of the in vitro and in vivo activities of IgG and F(ab')2 fragments of a mixture of three monoclonal anti-HER-2 antibdoies. *Clinical Cancer Research*, **10**, 3542–51.

Sporn, M.B. (1996) The war on cancer. *Lancet*, **347**, 1377–81.

Sprangers, M., Cull, A., Bjordal, K. *et al.* (1993) The European Organization for Research and Treatment of Cancer approach to quality of life assessment: Guidelines for developing questionnaire modules. *Quality of Life Research*, **2**, 287–95.

Sprent, J. (2003) Turnover of memory-phenotype CD8+ T cells. *Microbes and Infection*, **5**, 227–31.

Sprent, J. and Surh, C.D. (2003) Cytokines and T-cell homeostasis. *Immunology Letters*, **85**, 145–9.

Stacy, S., Krolick, K.A., Infante, A.J. and Kraig, E. (2002) Immunological memory and late onset autoimmunity *Mechanisms of Ageing and Development*, **123**, 975–85.

Stenman, U.H., Paus, E., Allard, W.J. *et al.* (1999) Summary report of the TD-3 workshop: characterization of 83 antibodies against prostate-specific antigen. *Tumour Biol*, **20**(Suppl 1),1–12.

Stieber, P., Aronsson, A.C., Bialk, P. *et al.* (1999) Tumor markers in lung cancer: EGTM recommendations. *Anticancer Res*, **19**, 2817–9.

Strachan, T. and Read, A.P. (1999) *Human Molecular Genetics 2*, BIOS Scientific Publishers, Oxford.

Strausberg, R.L. (2001) The Cancer Genome Anatomy Project: new resources for reading the molecular signatures of cancer. *J Pathol*, **195**(1), 31–40.

Strausberg, R.L., Buetow, K.H., Emmert-Buck, M.R., Klausner, R.D. (2000) The cancer genome anatomy project: building an annotated gene index. *Trends Genet*, **16**(3), 103–6.

Strausberg, R.L., Dahl, C.A., Klausner, R.D. (1997) New opportunities for uncovering the molecular basis of cancer. *Nat Genet*, **15** Spec No, 415–6.

Strauss, A. and Corbin, J., (1990) *Basics of Qualitative Research: Grounded Theory Procedures and Techniques*. Sage, California.

Sturgeon, C. (2002) Practice guidelines for tumor maker use in the clinic. *Clinical Chemistry*, **48**(8), 1151–9.

Sturgeon, C.M. (2001) Tumor markers in the laboratory: closing the guideline-practice gap. *Clin Biochem*, **34**, 353–9.

Sturgeon, C.M. and Seth, J. (1996) Why do immunoassays for tumour markers give differing results? – A view from the UK national external quality assessment schemes. *Eur J Clin Chem Biochem*, **34**, 755–9.

Sturgeon, C., Aronsson, A.C., Duffy, M.J. *et al.* (1999a) European group of tumour markers: Consensus recommendations. *Anticancer Research*, **19**, 2785–820.

Sturgeon, C., Dati, F., Duffy, M.J. *et al.* (1999b) Quality requirements and control: EGTM recommendations. *Anticancer Res*, **19**, 2791–4.

Summerhayes, M. and Daniels, S. (2003) *Practical Chemotherapy: A Multidisciplinary Guide*, Radcliffe Medical Press, Oxford.

Suresh, M.R. (2001) Cancer marker. In: *The Immunoassay Handbook* (ed Wild, D.), 2nd edn, Nature Publishing Group, pp. 635–63.

Sweep, C.G., Geurts-Moespot, J. (2000) EORT external quality assurance program for ER and PgR measurements: Trial 1998/1999. European organisation for research and treatment of cancer. *International Journal of Biological Markers*, **15**(1), 62–9.

Tagawa, M. (2000) Cytokine therapy for cancer. *Cancer Pharmaceutical Design*, **6**, 681–99.

Takahashi, S., Ito, Y., Hatake, K. and Sugimoto Y. (2006) Gene therapy for breast cancer. Review of clinical gene therapy trials for breast cancer and MDR1 gene therapy trial in Cancer Institute Hospital. *Breast Cancer*, **13**, 8–15.

Takeuchi T. (1995) Antitumour antibiotics discovered and studied at the institute of microbial chemistry. *J Cancer Res Clin Oncol*, **121**(9–10), 505–10.

TenBokkel Huinink, W., Lane, S.R., Ross, G.A. *et al.* (2004) Long term survival in a phase III randomised study of topotecan versus paclitaxel in advanced epithelial ovarian carcinoma. *Ann Oncol*, **15**(1), 100–3.

Thibodeau, J. and MacRae, J. (1997) Breast cancer survival: A phenomenological inquiry. *Advanced Nursing Science*, **19**(4), 65–74.

Thomas, C.M.G. and Sweep, C.G.J. (2001) Serum tumour markers: Past, state of art and future. *The International Journal of Biological Markers*, **16**(2), 73–85.

Thomas, J. and Retsas, A. (1999) Transacting self preservation: A grounded theory of the spiritual dimensions of people with terminal cancer. *International Journal of Nursing Studies*, **36**(3), 191–201.

Tiffany, R. (1998) *Oncology for Nurses and Healthcare Professionals: Diagnosis and Treatment*, vol **1**, 2nd edn, Harper & Row, London.

Tjoa, B.A., Erickson, S.J., Bowes, V.A. *et al.* (1997) Follow-up evaluation of prostate cancer patients infused with autologous dendritic cells pulsed with PSMA peptides. *The Prostate*, **32**, 272–8.

Tobinai, K. (2007) Antibody therapy for malignant lymphoma. *Intern Med*, **46**(2), 99–100.

Tortora, G.J. and Grabowski, S.R. (2003) *Principles of Anatomy and Physiology*, 10th edn, Harper Collins/Addison Wesley, New York, pp. 149–54.

Trask, B.J. (1991) Fluorescence in situ hybridization: applications in cytogenetics and gene mapping. *Trends Genet*, **7**(5), 149–54.

Tumor Marker Expert Panel (ASCO) (1996) Clinical practice guidelines for the use of tumor markers in breast and colorectal cancer. *J Clin Oncol*, **14**, 2843–77.

Tzioras, S., Pavlidis, N., Paraskevaidis, E. and Ioannidis, J.P. (2006) Effects of different chemotherapy regimens on survival for advanced cervical cancer: Systemic review and meta-analysis. *Cancer Treatment Review*, **33**, 24–38.

UICC (2002) *TNM Classification of Maligant Tumours*, Wiley-Liss, New York.

Valley, A.W. (2002) New treatment options for managing chemotherapy-induced neutropenia. *American Journal Health-System Pharmacy*, **15**(Suppl 4), S11–S16.

Van Cutsem, E., Twelves, C., Cassidy, J. *et al.* (2001) Oral capecitabine compared with intravenous fluorouracil plus leucovorin in patients with metatastic colorectal cancer: results of a large phase III study. *J Clin Oncol*, **19**(21), 4097–106.

Van der Zalm, J. and Bergum, V. (2000) Hermenutic-phenomenology: Providing living knowledge for nursing practice. *Journal of Advanced Nursing*, **31**(1), 211–8.

Van Manen, M. (1990) *Researching Lived Experience: Human Science for an Action Sensitive Pedagogy.* State University of New York Press, New York.

Van Oosterom, A.T., Mouridsen, H.T., Nielson, O.S. *et al.* (2002) Results of randomisd trials of the EORTC Soft Tissue and Bone Sarcoma Group (STBSG) with two different ifosfamide regimens in first and second line chemotherapy in advanced soft tissue sarcoma patients. *Eur J Cancer*, **38**(18), 2397–406.

Varmus, H.E. (1985) Viruses, genes, and cancer. I. The discovery of cellular oncogenes and their role in neoplasia. *Cancer*, **15**(55), 2324–8.

Venitt, S. (1978) The aetiology of human cancers. In: *Oncology for Nurses and Health Care Professionals, Vol 1, Pathology, Diagnosis and.Treatment* (ed P. Pritchard), Harper & Row, London.

Vial, T.and Descotes, J. (2003) Immunosuppressive drugs and cancer. *Toxicology*, **185**, 229–40.

Voet, D. and Voet, J.G. (1995) The expression and transmission of genetic information. In: *Biochemistry.* John Wiley and Sons, Inc., New York.

Vogelstein, B., Lane, D. and Levine AJ. (2000) Surfing the p53 network. *Nature*, **408**, 307–10.

Vogelzang, N.J., Rusthoven, J.J., Symanowski, J. *et al.* (2003) Phase III study of pemetrexed in combination with cisplatin versus cisplatin alone in patients with malignant pleural mesothelioma. *J Clin Oncol*, **21**(14), 2636–44.

Wacheck, V. and Zangemeister-Wittke, U. (2006) Antisense molecules for targeted cancer therapy. *Crit Oncol Hematol*, **59**(1), 65–73.

Wadman, M. (2006) The chips are down. *Nature*, **444**, 256–7.

Waldman, H. (2002) A personal history of Campath-1H antibody. *Medical Oncology*, **19**, S3–9.

Waldman, T.A. (2003) Immunmotherapy: Past, present and future. *Nature Medicine*, **9**(3), 269–77.

Walker, R.A. (2000) The significance of histological determination of HER-2 status in breast cancer. *The Breast*, **9**, 130–33.

Walter, J. (1977) Radiation hazards and protection: Cytotoxic chemotherapy. In: *Cancer and Radiotherapy: A short guide for nurses and medical students* (ed J. Walter), Churchill Livingstone, London.

Ward, R.L., Hawkins, N.J. and Smith, G.M. (1997) Unconjugated antibodies for cancer therapy: Lessons from the clinic. *Cancer Treatment Reviews*, **23**, 305–19.

Watson, J.D. and Crick, F.H.C. (1953) Molecular study of nucleic acids. *Nature*, **171**, 737–8.

Webb, N., Bottomley, M., Watson, C. and Brenchley, P. (1998) Vascular endothelial growth factor (VEGF) is released from platelets during blood clotting: implications for measurement of circulating VEGF levels in clinical disease. *Clin Sci*, **94**, 395–404.

Weber, B.L., Vogel, C. and Jones, S. *et al.* (1995) Intravenous vinorelbine as first-line and second line therapy in advanced breast cancer. *J Clin Oncol*, **13**(11), 2722–30.

Weiner, M.P. and Hudson, T.J. (2002) Introduction to SNPs: Discovery of markers for disease. *Biotechniques*, **10**(Suppl 4–7), 12–3.

Wells, M. (2001) The impact of cancer. In: *Cancer Nursing Care in Context* (eds J. Corner and C. Bailey), Blackwell Publising, Oxford.

West, H. (2003) *Introduction to Mill's Utilitarian Ethics*. Cambridge University Press, West Nyack, NY, USA.

Westgard, J.O., Barry, P.L., Hunt, M.R. and Groth, T. (1981) A multi-rule Shewhart chart for quality control in clinical chemistry. *Clin Chem*, **27**, 493–501.

Westgard, J.O. and Barry, P.L. (1986) *Improving Quality Control by Use of Multirule Control Procedures. Chapter 4 in Cost-Effective Quality Control: Managing the Quality and Productivity of Analytical Processes*. AACC Press, Washington, DC.

Wheeler, T. (2006) Psychological consequences of malignant melanoma: patients' experiences and preferences. *Nursing Standard*, **21**(10), 42–6.

White, S.C., Lorigan, P., Middleton, M.R. *et al.* (2001) Randomized phase II study of cyclophosphamide, doxorubicin and vincristine compared with single agent carboplatin in patients with poor prognosis small cell lung carcinoma. *Cancer*, **92**(3), 601–8.

Whittaker, J. (2001) Colorectal cancer. In: *Oncology Nursing in Practice* (ed J. Gabriel), Whurr Publishers, London.

Whittaker, J. and Sheppard, C. (2001) Body image and sexuality. In: *Oncology Nursing in Practice* (ed J. Gabriel), Whurr Publishers, London.

Widdice, L.E. and Kahn, J.A. (2006) Using the new HPV vaccines in clinical practice. *Cleveland Clinic Journal Medicine*, **73**(10), 929–35.

Wilkins, M.H.F., Stokes, A.R. and Wilson, H.R. (1953) Molecular structure of deoxypentose nucleic acids. *Nature*, **171**, 738–40.

Willett, W. (1989) The search for the cause of breast and colon cancer. *Nature*, **338**, 389–94.

Wilson, J., Connock, M., Sonq, F. *et al.* (2005) Imatinib for the treatment of patients with unresectable and/or metastatic gastrointestinal stromal tumours: systematic review and economic evaluation. *Health Technol Assess*, **9**(25), 1–142.

Wimpenny, P. and Gass, J. (2000) Interviewing in phenomenology and grounded theory: Is there a difference. *Journal of Advanced Nursing*, **31**(6), 1485–92.

Winter, G. and Milstein, C. (1991) Man-made antibodies. *Nature*, **349**, 293–9.

Wolfe, N. (1986) Neoplasia: Disorders of cell proliferation and differentiation. In: *Cell, Tissue and Disease: The Basis of Pathology*. Baillière Tindall, London.

Wood, P. (2006) *Understanding Immunology*, 2nd edn, Pearson Education, London.

World Health Organization (1994) Essential drugs for cancer chemotherapy. *Bull WHO*, **72**, 693–8.

World Medical Association, Declartion of Helsinki (2000) Ethical Principles for Medical Research Involving Human Subjects. (Accessed 16 July 2007).

www.bbcnews.co.uk/1/hi/London/England (Accessed 5 February 2007).

www.eurekalert.org.pub-release25th (Accessed January 2007).

Xiao, W. and Oefner, P.J. (2001) Denaturing high-performance liquid chromatography: A review. *Hum Mutat*, **17**(6), 439–74.

Yalow, R.S. and Berson, S.A. (1960) Immunoassay of endogenous plasma insulin in man. *J Clin Investig*, **39**, 1157–75.

Yang, X.D., Jia, X.C., Corvalan, J.R.F., Wang, P. and Deavis, G. (2001) Development of ABX-EGF, a fully human anti-EGF receptor monoclonal antibody, for cancer therapy. *Critical Reviews in Oncology/Hematology*, **38**, 17–23.

Yarbro, C., Frogge, M. and Goodman, M. (2005) *Cancer Nursing: Principles and Practice*, 6th edn, Jones and Bartlett Publishers, Boston, MA.

Young, C.D. and Feld, R. (2000) Approaches to the management of infections in cancer patients with neutropenia. In: *Textbook of Medical Oncology* (eds F. Cavalli, H.H. Hansen and S.B. Kaye), Martin Dunitz Ltd, London, pp. 565–81.

Young, W. (2001) Breaking bad news. In: *Oncology Nursing in Practice* (ed J. Gabriel), Whurr Publishers, London.

Zigmond, A. and Snaith, R. (1983) The Hospital Anxiety and Depression Scale. *Acta Psychiatr. Scand*, **67**, 361–70.

Zucker, S., Cao, J., Chen, W.T. *et al.* (2000) Critical appraisal of the use of matrix metalloproteinase inhibitors in cancer treatment. *Oncogene*, **19**(56), 6642–50.

Index

The Biology of Cancer, Second Edition.   Edited by J. Gabriel
© 2007 John Wiley & Sons, Ltd.

RC 262 .B47 2007

The biology of cancer